Intermittent Fasting
for Women Over 50

The Step-By-Step Guide to Reset the Metabolism, Losing Weight, Detox Your Body and Delay Aging. A New Healthy Lifestyle to Feeling at Your Best

Caren Cooper

TABLE OF CONTENTS

Introduction

Fasting intermittently is not a diet. It's an eating habit and a lifestyle. It's a way to prepare meals to ensure that someone gets the best out of them. Fasting Intermittently doesn't affect what you consume. It matters when you consume food. Intermittent fasting needs the body to be more self-productive and effective for it to work. Intermittent fasting typically implies that you intake the calories at a specific time and choose not to eat food for a longer time. Much research indicates that this form of living can provide benefits such as weight reduction, improved fitness, and enhanced lifespan. Experts claim that it's simpler to sustain an extended fasting regimen than conventional, calorie-controlled diets. Understanding the intermittent fasting of each person is different, and varying types will fit other individuals based on their needs.

Fasting intermittently is one of the best methods people have for reducing excess weight but holding healthy weight on, and it needs relatively least behavior modification. This is a positive idea because it ensures intermittent fasting fits under the easy enough task that one will simply do it, however significant enough that it can transform. Intermittent fasting shifts hormone levels to promote weight reduction.

In addition to reducing insulin in the bloodstream and increasing growth hormone levels, it enhances the production of the burning fat hormone known as noradrenaline or norepinephrine.

Studies suggest that a very effective method for weight reduction may be intermittent fasting. Short-term fasting can raise the body's metabolic rate by 3.6 to 14 percent due to these hormones' changes. By encouraging one to eat less, and burn additional calories, by manipulating all calorie calculation aspects, intermittent fasting induces weight loss.

In contrast to other weight loss trials, a review study showed that this eating style would induce 3 to 8 percent weight loss from 3 to 24 weeks, which is a significant change. There is no each-size-fits-all approach when it comes to intermittent fasting at the end of the day. The one approach that you should hold on to in the long term is the right pattern with proper nutrition for you.

Chapter 1

What Is Intermittent Fasting?

Intermittent fasting is nothing but fasting for extended periods and eating only within an allowed window of time. So, what does fasting do and how does it help you lose weight?

Feeding and Fasting

Our body is continuously in one of two states, which are the feeding or fasting states. When we eat a meal, our body is in the feeding state and it remains in this state for the next 4 to 5 hours. We do not feel hungry in this state. After about 6 to 8 hours comes the post-feeding state or the intermediate state, where we may or may not feel hungry. The body uses our most recent meal to gather energy when needed for some action. After this comes the fasting stage, which lasts until we have another meal.

We haven't taken a meal during this fasting stage, and our body has already used the last meal to derive energy. Now it turns to our stored energy reserves, which are the fats in our body. This is the stage when fats get burned. In this stage, we feel hungry and our body looks for food to use as fuel, but not finding any recent meal, because we haven't eaten, burns our fat stores. This is why fasting has been known to be such a meaningful way to burn accumulated fats. But if we have provided our body with food, it doesn't enter the fasting stage and no fat gets burned and our body resorts to our next meal for energy.

The Science behind Intermittent Fasting

To understand how intermittent fasting works, it is essential to understand what usually happens in our bodies with the food we eat. Whenever we take a meal, eat or even drink something, our body releases a hormone called insulin. Insulin is widely popular as a medicine given to people with diabetes. Still, not much thought is given to it as to the why and the how of it.

This insulin released at the time of food consumption acts as the monitor of our blood glucose levels. Insulin takes care of the amount of glucose we need immediately as energy for our actions. It decides how much of this glucose should be converted to glycogen, which is nothing but a readily available energy source, and how much of it should be stored as fat for later use. This is the reason why insulin is also known as a fat-storing hormone. Some people with diabetes cannot have this glucose monitor in their blood and hence need external insulin injections to handle their blood glucose levels.

If you are frequently or regularly eating, then your body is regularly releasing insulin. This leads to more and more storage of energy in the form of fats. Your body has no chance to reach your already present fat reserves to burn them for energy; instead, it continually adds to them. One important thing to keep in mind is keeping your insulin levels in check, which can be easily done by adequately scheduling your meals.

Ghrelin is known as the hunger hormone as this is the hormone responsible for causing us hunger and pushing us to eat more. Suppose your regular eating schedule involves three meals a day. In that case, your body secretes the ghrelin hormone at your three mealtimes to signal it is time to eat. Ghrelin release does not necessarily mean your body needs food, it merely means it is your regular eating time and your body reminds you to eat. You can regulate ghrelin levels by intermittent fasting so that your body gets adjusted to your new eating schedules.

Leptin is another important hormone that helps regulate your food intake. It is also called the satiety hormone, because it signals that you have had enough food and hints to you to stop eating. It helps you feel full and satisfied. The higher the leptin levels the less likely you are to eat food. Naturally, since birth, we are wired to have a balance of both ghrelin and leptin levels. Our ever-changing lifestyles and unhealthy food practices, causes this inherent balance to be disturbed. These hormone levels swing, either way, causing us to put on more weight through unregulated eating habits.

You see the best demonstration of the working of these hormones in infants and toddlers to some extent. Children in these age groups have their minds off when they would like to eat and how much. This is their hormones talking and they are often doing a better job than us to keep our food intake in check. We often see parents struggling to feed their toddlers, running around the house or the backyard trying to get a few bites in. The thing is, a toddler generally doesn't eat when they are full. Their leptin tells them they have had enough, and they refuse to eat more. We, as concerned parents, sometimes force them to eat. Here begins the imbalance of these hormones. Leptin no longer functions appropriately, because we seem to eat even when it signals us not to. Right from that age, we begin to tell our brains we eat at certain times, or because we have food on hand, or we have something before us that we absolutely cannot pass up. This messes up the hormone signals. We are not eating like we used to in the infant to toddler age, when we are hungry; instead, we eat because it is our supposed mealtime, even if we do not feel the need. All three hormones, insulin, ghrelin, and leptin, are now in quite an imbalanced state, leading us to feel hungry all the time, causing us to eat all the time, thereby increasing our fat storage.

The Wrong Approach

In most diets, the most popular phenomenon is to divide your whole food intake per day into six or more small portions. These meals are taken throughout the day with a gap of a few hours in between. It has been a popular belief for quite some time now that doing so helps your metabolism and helps reduce weight because you aren't feeding on large quantities at once. Instead, what this truly does is keeps your insulin levels always high. What this does in turn is convert all the digested sugars into fats.

Naturally in a single day, you wouldn't require all the energy that even six small meals could give you. So, the sugar monitor in your blood, insulin, directs all the unused sugars to be turned into fat and stored for later. Doing this day in and day out, every day, simply increases your fat stores. We need to use up the already stored fat not add more to it. But that is precisely what eating several small meals in a day does. Only when we give our body time to reduce its insulin levels in the blood will it be able to access the stored fat and use that for energy. This is impossible when a constant food intake is going on. The time intervals between these small meals are too short to induce our bodies to access the stored fat, because it still has the glucose from the most recent meal to make use of.

Therefore, contrary to popular belief, six or more small meals are the wrong way to go about it. The need of the hour is to look for something that gives your body sufficient time to reach those stored fats and burn them, and intermittent fasting is ideal for just that!

Drawbacks of Intermittent Fasting for Women Over 50

Intermittent fasting has a few drawbacks, especially in the beginning stages, when a person is still getting accustomed to retimed eating schedules. These drawbacks are few. For women, who can and cannot apply intermittent fasting schedules, we should decide based on their medical and physical conditions, which we shall look at later on in the book. But once a woman has decided and begun fasting, it is only a matter of adjusting and adapting oneself to the new eating patterns. Whatever disadvantages or drawbacks arise due to intermittent fasting, all stem from this adjustment stage.

Severe hunger pangs, lightheadedness, dizziness, dehydration, headaches, and muscle weakness are problems that people usually face due to intermittent fasting schedules. These are also restricted to the adapting or adjusting stage. One rare drawback of the fasting system is infertility. But this is hardly an issue after a couple of weeks of stopping the schedule and less so for women over 50 who are mostly beyond the child-bearing age.

Several specific types of intermittent fasting.

The most prominent ones include

- The 16:8 method
- The warrior diets
- Time-restricted fasting
- Eat stop eat
- Spontaneous meal skipping
- The 5:2 diet
- Alternate-day fasting (ADF)

All intermittent fasting methods are beneficial and effective, but it depends on the individual to find out which works better.

Types of Intermittent Fasting

16/8 Intermittent Fasting Method

One of the most favored forms of fasting for losing weight is the 16/8 intermittent fasting plan. Often, it's called time-restricted fasting, though some variants are subtly different. A person fasts for 16 hours in the 16:8 model and restricts eating to an 8-hour window of time. As a portion of the 16-hour window, several individuals miss breakfast. So, for instance, you could eat during the 12 pm to 8 pm range.

Some people, though, choose to miss supper instead. You could restrict the eating window to 9 am & 5 pm per day with this. To eat calories, a person can pick up every 8-hour time and miss dinner or breakfast.

You might still eat the main meal a day for this fasting pattern. One can choose the timing of meals, like breakfast at 10:00 am, lunch will be at 2:00 pm, and dinner at 5:30 pm. By 6:00 pm, a person can finish eating their dinner so that all of the food consumption is done inside the 10 am to 6 pm window, which is eight hours.

Fasting limits the consumption of calorie-containing drinks and food to a limited window of 8 hours a day. For the rest of the 16 hours of each day, it involves refraining from food. Whereas other diet plans can set rigid rules and regulations, the 16/8 process is more flexible and based on the time-restricted feeding (TRF) method.

This fasting model may help one lose weight and lower blood pressure by limiting the number of hours that one can eat throughout the day. A review study found that the 16/8 technique helped decrease body fat and maintained muscle mass in several participants when coupled with physical exercise. A much more recent study showed that the 16/8 method did not hinder muscle gains in women performing aerobic exercise.

While the 16/8 technique can easily fit into every lifestyle, it may be difficult for some individuals to avoid eating 16 hours straight. Additionally, the potential benefits associated with 16/8 intermittent fasting can be negated by eating junk food or too many snacks during the 8-hour window. To maximize this intermittent fasting's health benefits, make sure to eat a healthy, balanced diet containing fresh vegetables, fruits, whole grains, good lean protein, and healthy fats.

The 5:2-Method of Intermittent Fasting

The 5:2 diet usually entails consuming normal amounts of calories to five days each week while reducing your calorie consumption for only 2 days of the week to 500-600 calories. Also known as the Fast Diet, this diet was popularized by British journalists. The 5:2 diet is a simple and direct intermittent fasting plan. You normally eat 5 days a week and don't limit your calories but also do not eat fried or unhealthy snacks. Then, you drop the calorie consumption to one-quarter of your standard requirements for the remaining 2 days of the same week. This means reducing the calorie intake to just 500 calories each day, 2 days per week, for someone who regularly consumes 2,000 calories each day.

According to research, for people with type 2 diabetes, the 5:2 diet is as efficient as daily calorie reduction for weight loss and blood sugar control. Another study showed that the 5:2 diet for both weight reduction and the treatment of metabolic disorders such as cardiac failure and diabetes was almost as successful as constant calorie restriction.

As the person gets to select the days they are fasting, the 5:2 diet promises versatility, and there are no guidelines on whether or what to consume on full-calorie days. Having said that, it should be remembered that eating "usually" on full-calorie days does not grant you a free pass to consume anything you want.

It's not convenient to restrict oneself to only 500 calories a day, even though it's just 2 days a week. And, you can feel sick or faint from eating very few calories. The 5:2 diet might be efficient, but it's not for everybody. To see if the 5:2 diet could be appropriate for you, speak to the doctor. There are days for low-calorie, and you can eat around 25% of the calorie requirements, typically about 500 to 750 calories per day, and are sometimes referred to as "modified fasts."

It is recommended that women consume 500 calories on fasting days, and men consume 600. You can consume 2 regular meals of 250 calories per woman for two fasting days and 300 calories per man. No trials are evaluating the 5:2 diet itself, as opponents rightly point out, but there are loads of studies about the advantages of intermittent fasting.

Low Carb Group 5:2 Intermittent Fasting has slightly larger decreases in insulin resistance and insulin relative to the low-calorie regular group. This category contained the most persons who had lost nearly 5% of their body weight.

Low Carb Group with Fat and Protein Intermittent Fasting 5:2: lowered insulin and insulin resistance almost the same as the low-calorie regular group. This category has the lowest amount of weight reduction that came from fat. It makes sense as protein will try to stop fat-burning (ketosis).

Furthermore, cholesterol levels, blood pressure, and inflammation were decreased for both classes. All intermittent fasting groups lost more body fat than the normal calorie restriction community. The investigators concluded that the IF 5:2 diet of fewer than 40 grams of carbohydrates a day produced better outcomes of the three diets for body fat reduction and insulin sensitivity improvement.

Alternate-Day Intermittent Fasting

As the title suggests, every other day, alternate-day intermittent fasting is when someone fast or severely limits their caloric intake. For alternate-day fasting, a person fasts every other day. The alternative fasting method of every other day is much less popular. Furthermore, trying it is perhaps the most difficult form of intermittent fasting. This fasting routine may not be feasible. As per the review study, it may lead to intense hunger on fasting days. This other analysis revealed that most people who could do intermittent fasting were the respondents who tried to do alternative day fasting to lose weight. It also did not generate greater weight loss or maintenance of weight. Usually, this intermittent fasting is not strongly recommended. For the whole day, it is difficult not to eat. The person should worry about their blood sugar, levels of insulin, and energy. Your ability to think can also be disturbed. You are going to be extremely hungry.

A professor of nutrition popularized this strategy. This fast consists of 25 % of one's calorie and need almost 500 calories. On non-fasting days are typical eating days, people could fast every other day. This is a common approach to weight loss. In reality, alternative day fasting has been seen to help obese people who want to lose excessive weight. By two weeks, the adverse effects (like extreme hunger) diminished, and by four weeks, the participants continued to become more comfortable with the diet. The drawback of that during the experiment's eight weeks, respondents said they never really felt their stomachs were full, which can make it difficult to adhere to this fasting method.

This intermittent fasting has several different versions. During intermittent fasting days, a few of them allow almost 500 calories. Some versions of this technique were used in many studies showing the positive effects of intermittent fasting. A complete fast may seem far more extreme every other day, so it is not suggested for beginners. You can go to bed quite hungry several times a week with this method, that is not pleasant at all and, in the long term, probably unsustainable.

9

24-Hour fast/ One Meal a Day

Between meals, the trick is to fast for 24 hours. Eat at 7 pm on the first day, for example, and fast until 7 pm the following day. Conversely, a person can choose to eat earlier, either lunch or breakfast, and fast until the next day for 24 hours. The concept is that every day you eat a meal but allow your body to fast for a longer period. This sort of fasting is usually performed once or twice a week, but it can be more frequently adopted. This type of fasting is not for everyone.

The OMAD intermittent fasting (one meal a day) is when one limits their eating window to only 1 hour per day, and for the remaining 23 hours, fasting happens. This is the ultimate type of intermittent fasting, and for many individuals, it can be an effective strategy for extreme weight loss.

Some of the risk factors of cardiovascular disease can be eased by this type of intermittent fasting but under strict medical supervision. During that window, one has to be able to last 23 hours without meals and resist the temptation to eat, as extreme hunger is a common complication of this sort of fasting.

Eat-Stop-Eat

Eat Stop Eat is an unorthodox approach to intermittent fasting popularized by an "Eat Stop Eat" journalist. This intermittent fasting plan includes classifying one or two non-consecutive days each week for a 24-hour cycle. During which one abstains from eating or fasting. one can eat freely during the remaining days of the week, but eating a well-rounded diet and avoiding overconsumption is suggested.

The reason behind a 24-hour fast every week is that eating fewer calories will ultimately lead to weight loss. Fasting for 24 hours can result in a metabolic shift that causes one's body to utilize stored fat rather than glucose as an energy source. But it requires a huge amount of self-discipline to avoid food for 24 hours on end and may lead to bingeing and excessive consumption later on. It may also result in eating disordered patterns.

To identify this pattern's potential health benefits and weight loss properties, much research is required regarding the Eat Stop Eat diet. Before attempting Eat Avoid Eat, speak with the doctor, and see if that could be an appropriate weight reduction solution for you. This strategy varies from other plans in that it emphasizes flexibility.

The Warrior diets

This intermittent fasting plan is called the warrior diet based on ancient warriors' eating patterns. The Warrior Diet, which was created in 2001, is a bit more dramatic than the 16:8 techniques but less rigid than Eat Stop Eats method. It comprises eating almost nothing or very little during the day for 20 hours, then eating as much food as desired at night in a 4-hour eating window.

During the 20-hour fast period, the Warrior Diet promotes people to consume small quantities of hard-boiled eggs, dairy products, vegetables, and raw fruits and fluids with no calories. After the 20-hour fast, in a 4-hour eating window, individuals can eat anything they want, but it must be unprocessed. Organic foods and healthy are suggested. Although there is no research, especially on the Warrior Diet, studies show that time-restricted eating cycles can lead to weight loss.

There could be many other health advantages of time-restricted feeding periods. Studies indicate that feeding cycles that are time-restricted can inhibit diabetes, limit the development of tumors, postpone aging, and improve lifespan. More research on the Warrior Diet is needed to grasp its weight-loss advantages fully.

It can be challenging to adopt the Warrior Diet since it reduces significant calorie intake to only 4 hours a day. Excessive consumption of calories at night is a widespread problem. The Warrior Diet can often result in disordered eating habits. Speak to the doctor if you feel up to the warrior diet's task to see if it's correct for you. During the day, it means consuming tiny quantities of fresh fruits and vegetables and eating one big meal at night. Within a four-hour eating window, you fast throughout the day and dine at night. One of the first common diets to incorporate a form of intermittent fasting was the Warrior Diet.

This lifestyle's food preference is fairly close to that of the paleo diet, mainly unprocessed foods, and whole foods. The Warrior Diet supports only tiny quantities of veggies and fruits to thrive throughout the day, then consume a big meal at night.

Spontaneous Meal Skipping

To enjoy any of its advantages, you don't need to adopt a formal intermittent fasting schedule. Another choice is to miss meals from time - to - time, such as cooking and eating and not consuming them when you are too busy or don't feel hungry. It's a misconception that every few hours, people ought to consume calories before they enter hunger mode or lose their muscles. Your body is well prepared to cope with long stretches of hunger, let alone the loss of one to two meals from time to time.

Therefore, one day you just don't feel hungry, miss breakfast, and only have a good lunch or dinner. Or, if you're going anywhere and you can't seem to find something you want to consume, do it easily and momentarily. It's simply a random, sporadic quick-to-miss one or two meals anytime you are tempted to do so. Only make sure during the other meals to consume nutritious foods.

Choose-Your-Day Fasting

This is more of an adventure of your own choice. Every other day or once or twice each week, you could do time-restricted fasting as you fast for 16 hours, and to eat for eight hours it means that Saturday could be a normal eating day, and by 8 p.m. one would stop eating; then at noon on Sunday, the eating will be resumed. It's like skipping breakfast several days a week.

Time-Restricted Fasting

You pick a feeding window every day with this form of Intermittent fasting, which will ideally leave a 14 to 16-hour fasting window. It is recommended for women over 50 to fast for no more than 14 hours each day due to hormonal issues. Fasting encourages autophagy, as discussed before, the simple and healthy cellular housekeeping process in which the body clears degenerated protein, cell debris, and other things that hinder the way of mitochondrial health, which begins when the body's glycogen is depleted, experts say. Doing it could help maximize the metabolism of fat cells and help optimize the function of insulin.

For this to work, a person may set their eating window from 9 a.m. To 5 p.m. This can work particularly well for somebody with a family who is still eating an early dinner. Far too much of the time spent fasting is still time spent asleep. Depending on that, when a person sets their eating window, they won't miss any meals. But this depends on how consistent one can be. If your schedule is very flexible, or you want the freedom to go out now and then for breakfast, or you want late dinners, it may not be for you to have daily fasting cycles.

Choosing Your Intermittent Fasting Plan

You may use a standard method that limits daily eating to a span of six to eight hours per day. For example, one may decide to try fasting for 16/8, eat for eight hours, and fast for 16 hours. Many experts are supporters of the daily regimen: in the long run, most individuals find it convenient to adhere to this easy pattern.

Another approach is the 5:2 strategy, which includes eating five days a week regularly. One may restrict themselves to a daily 500 to 600-calorie meal for the rest of the two days.

Longer stretches without food are not inherently healthier for someone new to intermittent fasting, like 24, 36, 48, and 72-hour fasting periods, and can be risky. Going too long without eating could promote the body to start storing more fat in reaction to hunger and malnourishment.

Research suggests that intermittent fasting will take two to four weeks until the body becomes used to it. As you're becoming accustomed to the new schedule, you may feel hungry or grumpy. But, it says, study participants who make it past the time of transition prefer to adhere to the program, and they find that they feel healthier.

In deciding which intermittent fasting method is the best for you, your tolerance of hunger pangs can direct you. Although intermittent fasting for most active adults is usually safe, it is not intended for everybody.

Chapter 2

The Relationship Between Intermittent Fasting and Reproductive Hormones

One way in which fasting affects reproductive hormones is due to the hypothalamic-pituitary-gonadal combination in both women and men. This is, thankfully, more commonly referred to as the HPG axis. In daily spurts, the hypothalamus releases the gonadotropin-releasing hormone (GnRH), called "pulses."

GnRH pulses instruct the pituitary gland to release follicular stimulating hormone (LH) and luteinizing hormone (LH) (FSH).

Then, LH and FSH function on the gonads. In women, estrogen and progesterone production that we need to release a mature egg is stimulated by LH and FSH.

In males, they stimulate testosterone and sperm production. Because this chain of reactions occurs in women on a very specific, regular cycle, GnRH pulses need to be accurately timed, or everything can get out of whack. Eggs have not been published, and cycles have ended.

In some women, also short-term fasting, say, three days may change these hormonal pulses. There is also some evidence that skipping a single meal will start to put our hormonal system on alert, which of course, is not an emergency by itself. This may be why some women run into intermittent fasting issues.

But why does eating less put alertness in our bodies? For many years, scientists thought that a woman's body fat percentage regulated her reproductive system; if fat reserves fell below a certain amount, hormones became confused and the cycle stopped around 11 percent.

Boom: no possibility of conception

This has made a lot of sense from an evolutionary perspective. Our ancestors, who did not have access to Costco and Amazon, would be of major concern to have a low food supply. (Read: It wouldn't be a good time to give birth or raise young people.) So, if you were to lose body fat, your body might think that there's not much to eat and try to escape reproduction. But the matter is more complex than that. Even before body fat drops, female bodies tend to go on alert.

Consequently, women who are not particularly lean can stop ovulating and lose their periods, too. That is why scientists now suspect that the overall energy balance may be more important for this process than the percentage of body fat, how many calories you eat compared to how many you burn.

How your diet can work against you, and too much stress

You are known to be in a negative energy balance when you consistently consume less energy than you expend. How you lose weight is how you get into a negative energy balance. So, this is exactly what many people are trying to accomplish by dieting. But in the context of other stressors, when it is extreme or goes on for too long, it is the cause of the hormonal spiral that is seen in some women on an empty stomach. Not only does negative energy equilibrium result from eating less food.

Also, it can result from:

- Poor nutrition
- An excessive amount of exercise
- Too much stress
- Infection, disease, chronic inflammation
- Too little rest and recovery
- Heck, by attempting to keep warm, we can even use up energy.

It may be enough for any combination of stressors to bring you into an unnecessary negative energy balance and avoid ovulation.

For instance:

- too many days at the gym and not eating enough vegetables and fruits nursing flu and training for a marathon
- You may be thinking, 'Did she just reference paying the mortgage?'

In harming your hormonal health, psychological stress may play a part.
Our bodies can't say the difference between our thoughts and feelings created by a real threat and something theoretical. (Such as thinking about how to get your abs.)

These "threats may increase our levels of the stress hormone cortisol." And with cortisol? It inhibits GnRH, our old friend.

Fast reminder: GnRH disruption causes a cascade effect that can inhibit the development of estrogen and progesterone hormones essential for reproduction in your ovaries.

So, you might be hovering at 30% fat. But if you are in a negative energy balance for too long a period, especially if you're very stressed, reproduction stops.

Why does intermittent fasting impact the hormones of women more than those of men?

We aren't completely sure

When your partner walks around looking wispy after practicing intermittent fasting for a few months, we know it is not an easy thing to learn.

But there are several possible explanations for contributing:

1. Women may be more sensitive than men to changes in nutrient equilibrium.
When fasting or significantly restricting calories, men and women seem to respond differently. This may be due to kisspeptin, a molecule similar to a protein vital in the reproductive process. Kisspeptin stimulates the production of GnRH in both sexes, and we understand that it is very susceptible to leptin, insulin, and ghrelin-hormones that control and respond to feelings of hunger and fullness.

Females have more kisspeptin than males, interestingly. More kisspeptin may indicate that women's bodies are more susceptible to energy balance changes. Fasting more readily causes women's production of kisspeptin to dip compared to men. It tosses GnRH off kilter12 when kisspeptin drops, which upsets the entire monthly hormonal cycle.

2. Compared with men, restricting certain nutrients such as protein may also have different effects on women.
Women tend to eat less protein than men in general and women who eat quickly usually eat even less protein (because they eat less overall). That's an issue because protein provides amino acids that are critical for the process of reproduction. If amino acids get too low. If the uterus's lining does not thicken, it is impossible to implant an egg, and pregnancy cannot occur.

Hence, low-protein diets can reduce fertility. Throughout our bodies, we have estrogen receptors, including in our hearts, GI tract and bones. Adjust the estrogen balance. Throughout this debate, you adjust metabolic functions: cognition, mood, digestion, regeneration, protein turnover, bone formation, appetite, and energy balance may be most important. Estrogens alter the peptides in the brain stem that tell you to feel full (cholecystokinin) or hungry (ghrelin). Estrogens also stimulate neurons in the hypothalamus that halt the production of peptides that regulate appetite.

Do something that causes your estrogen to reduce (like fast), and you might feel a lot hungrier than you would under normal circumstances, and eat a lot more.

Oestrogen affects the storage of fat, too. Oestrogens are vital metabolic regulators, as you can see. Yes, plural, estrogenic. Three different estrogen types found in the body are estriol, estradiol, and estrone, also known as estrogenic metabolites. Over time, the proportions of these Oestrogens change. Estradiol is the major player before menopause. But estradiol drops after menopause, whereas estrone stays about the same. It remains unclear the exact roles of each of these estrogens. But some theorize that a decrease in estradiol may cause an increase in the storage of fat.

The theory does not, however, explain anything. Although a decrease in estradiol may be associated with an increase in fat storage, it is probably not the only cause. Increased fat around menopause is often caused by aging, reduced muscle mass, and appetite changes; more generally, low estradiol is also associated with higher appetite). So intermittent fasting in women for weight loss... is complicated. Because... Women's bodies could just be more susceptible to energy balance shifts.

And...

It can disturb the HPG axis when our bodies' sense shifts and our whole hormonal cycle is thrown away. If other stressors are wasting our resources, this hormonal turmoil can be exacerbated further.

Intermittent fasting can minimize estrogen, and reduced estrogen can improve the storage of appetite and fat. So, fasting to control your weight? Maybe it's kind of... counterproductive. The more you struggle, the harder it gets, like being caught in one of those Chinese finger traps.

Intermittent Fasting and Lifetime of Females

Women, childbearing or not, go through many different stages of existence, marked by major hormonal alterations.

Such hormonal changes can have major physical and psychological impacts and affect sleep, digestion, reactivity to stress, and metabolism. Here are a couple of those stages and how they may be affected by intermittent fasting.

Intermittent Fasting in Girls and Teens

Fasting is not recommended during times of intense development, including childhood and adolescence. Many kids are born with the ability to monitor their food consumption reasonably well, provided they are given a variety of healthy choices to choose from.

Teenagerhood (and even earlier) may be a time of extreme self-scrutiny and social comparison and is often considered "dieting" by many young girls. It is a sensitive time, even when it is necessary to change eating habits. Focus on growing appetite awareness and conscious eating, and prioritizing whole, nutritious foods instead of restricting food. Promoting an enjoyable, stress-free relationship with food and a kind, compassionate relationship with the body as much as possible.

Intermittent Ovulation and Fasting

Intermittent fasting might make things complicated if you're trying to conceive. Ovulation can be inhibited by fasting. No egg is released if you're not ovulating. It can't be fertilized if no egg gets released. Doctors or other health practitioners may have advised certain women to lose weight before becoming pregnant. Many women are starting to think more critically about their health while contemplating pregnancy and view weight loss as a step in this direction.

Whatever the justification for considering intermittent fasting, remember this for hormonal equilibrium, intermittent fasting is not the right protocol for weight loss to suggest for most women. Most women do well with moderate, sustainable, good eating behaviors in the reproductive phase of life. Unless a woman is paid to look or act in a certain way (such as a physical competitor or a professional athlete), it may not be worth sacrificing fertility and hormonal balance.

Intermittent Fasting during Pregnancy

Pregnancy is like childhood and adolescence, a period of intense development. Weight gain is a desirable consequence of developing pregnancy and is a symbol of a stable, growing infant. Even though weight gain is needed during this period, the upward-creeping scale makes many women uncomfortable. During this time, women who are extremely body-conscious or want to lose weight before pregnancy can also think about weight loss.

Some women may also be recommended to control their weight during pregnancy by a doctor. (Which is a lot to ask when you feel nauseous and exhausted and anxious about changing, you know, your entire life.) Even if a medical professional proposes weight loss, fasting during this period is not suitable.

Focus on increasing nutrition instead of limiting food: striving to get sufficient healthy fats ,protein, quality, colorful vegetables, carbohydrates and fruits. (And if you can just eat bread and pickles from your topsy-turvy stomach, that's great...) You can also boost your health and control weight gain by exercising, given that your doctor has cleared you. We have an infographic for that too if you're curious about what to do: how to exercise during pregnancy.

Intermittent Fasting Breastfeeding

If you have a baby and decide to breastfeed, you already know that this is a difficult time for your body: you have yet to recover from giving birth, you are probably sleep-deprived, and you have turned your whole life upside down. Plus, the baby is now treating you like a buffet of all-you-can-drinks. Your body requires extra nurturing, extra nutrients, and less stress during this time. For these reasons, for breastfeeding women, intermittent fasting is probably not a good protocol.

Many moms worry about "losing the weight of the baby" and may feel pressured and impatient to get back their "pre-baby" body. Try moderate exercise and portion management for safe, sustainable weight loss.

Intermittent Fasting in Ageing Females

Puberty, menstruation, perhaps pregnancy, and postpartum. Just what a rollercoaster.

Then comes menopause, another hormonal transition point that can disrupt women's lives physically and socially and psychologically. After decades of being dedicated to children, spouses, and careers, women may return to themselves in this phase. Or they may be busier than ever before, looking after aging parents and young adult children.

(The one who's just. Won't. Move. Out.) Increasing age often triggers a desire to concentrate on health, whatever the context.

Because of its association with longevity, some women are interested in intermittent fasting. In an uncomplicated way, others just want to lose fat. While we do not have quality science on whether intermittent fasting is beneficial to menopausal or postmenopausal women, we know that it is also a stressor to restrict food.

Women who are concerned with controlling body weight control food intake tend to have higher levels of cortisol than women who do not. Connect that to the sleep disturbances that are so normal in menopause, and your "stress bucket" gets pretty full. Lower levels of estrogen also mean that your body has a reduced ability to cope with stress. That bucket is filling up faster than it used to be. Although many stressors, such as exercise, learning, and change, are good for us, they only make us stronger if we permit ourselves to recover from them.

So, if you're a woman in this phase, try intermittent fasting only if:

- You're getting quality sleep.
- Your stress is low.
- You don't have any nutrient deficiencies.
- You are not tormented by hot flashes and mood swings.

So, for women, is intermittent fasting bad?

All right, not necessarily.

Surely, however, fasting is not for everyone. And the truth is some women are not even supposed to bother experimenting.

Do not attempt intermittent fasting if:

- You are pregnant
- You have a history of eating disorders.
- You're under chronic stress
- You're not sleeping well.
- You're new to exercise and diet.

Pregnant women have additional energy requirements. So, if you start a family, it's not a good idea for intermittent fasting. Ditto if you have chronic stress or if you don't sleep well. Your body requires nurturing, not extra stress. And if you've suffered in the past, you probably understand that a fasting regimen could lead you down a path that could cause more problems for you.

Are there any benefits for women from intermittent fasting?

Based on what we observe, if the body sees it as a major stressor, intermittent fasting potentially affects reproductive health. Your overall health and fitness are affected by something that affects your reproductive health. And if you're not planning on having any biological children. However, intermittent protocols of fasting differ, with some being far more severe than others. And variables such as your age, your dietary status, the amount of time you are fasting, and other stressors in your life, including exercise, are also likely to be important.

The Perfect Women's Intermittent Fasting Schedule

There are several ways of dipping your toe in if you ever want to try intermittent fasting.

Given how much remains unknown, instead of diving into advanced intermittent fasting, a cautious approach is probably safer. For a few days, you could start by keeping a food journal. Get a sense of what you eat, how much, and how often you eat it.

Do you eat late at night and have snacks during the day? Do your servings, or do you prefer lighter meals, seem to be large and fill you up? Do you get protein for every meal? Huh? Veggies?

"You should experiment with intermittent fasting "lite" once you have some more knowledge of your baseline. Here are a few ways to do that.

Start by stretching the interval between eating. What happens when you stop, if you normally snack between meals? Are you feeling greedy, dizzy, and mad? Does starvation ebb and flow? Do you feel totally fine? Try to extend the time between your last meal in the evening and the next morning for your first meal. For instance, if you usually eat your last meal at 8 p.m. and then eat breakfast at 7 a.m. (11 a.m. fasting), try to eat your last meal at 6 p.m. and eat breakfast at 8 or 10 a.m. a little later (fasting 14-16 hours).

As you attempt these experiments, continue to physically check-in with yourself:

Although you may be a little bit more uncomfortable than usual, is the hunger manageable overall? Or do you notice that even now?

- Are you more or less reactive when stress spikes?
- What is your sleep like?
- Your drive for sex?
- Your levels of energy?
- Your workout performance?

Often check in with your thoughts about food and your body:

- Do you feel embarrassed or ashamed if you have to break early on the fast?
- Do you feel deprived and so overeat when it is permissible to eat?
- Do you feel hypercritical about the shape of your body or tie sentiments of meaning to how fine you are IF-ing?

Track yourself with curiosity, compassion, and integrity.

If you're feeling mentally sharp, and energetic, and all systems are normal, proceed with a gentle intermittent fasting method, or try extending the fasting window a little further.

When to avoid intermittent fasting

If you're feeling obsessive, unhinged, and chronically lethargic, ease off.

Stop intermittent fasting if:

- your menstrual cycle ceases or becomes erratic
- you have trouble falling asleep
- hair starts to fall out more than normal
- you start to grow dry skin or acne
- you're finding you don't recover from workouts as quickly
- your injuries are slow to heal
- Declines in the stress tolerance
- Your mood begins to swing.

- Your heart begins to go pitter-patter oddly.
- Your interest in romance fizzles (and when it does, your lady parts stop appreciating it),
- Your digestion slows down considerably,
- It still seems like you feel cold.
- Add some snacks, and/or reduce to 12 hours or less your nightly fasting time.

Don't get caught up in doing it right." There are many ways to change bodies, as we've learned from coaching more than 100,000 clients, and none of those approaches requires you to be flawless.

What to do if it isn't for you to fast

When you think intermittent fasting isn't a good fit, how do you get in shape and lose weight?

Know the fundamentals of outstanding eating.

Fasting or not, concentrating on meal quality does not go wrong: prioritize lean proteins, colorful vegetables, and fruits, healthy fats, and quality carbohydrates. Crowd out snacks, caloric drinks, and foods that are refined. Cook and eat food in its entirety. Regularly workout. Remain consistent. (And if you want any help doing all this, recruit a coach.)

These simple elements are critical to your health and well-being. Sure, it may be common for intermittent fasting. Yet women are different than men, and there are different needs in our bodies.

Best Types of Intermittent Fasting for Women

When it comes to dieting, no one strategy applies to everyone equally; In the case of intermittent fasting, this is even more true. Women should usually take a more relaxed approach to fast than men.

This can include shorter periods of fasting, fewer days of fasting, and/or a limited number of calories expended on days of fasting.

Here are some of the best kinds of women's intermittent fasting:

- Crescendo Method: Fasting for two or three days a week for 12-16 hours. Fasting days in the week should be non-consecutive and uniformly spaced (for example, Monday, Wednesday, and Friday).

- Eat-stop-eat (also referred to as the 24-hour protocol): Once or twice a week, a complete 24-hour fast: (maximum of two times a week for women). Start with fasting for 14-16 hours and build up gradually.

- The 5:2 diet (also called "The Fast Diet"): Limit calories for two days a week to 25 % of your usual consumption (about 500 calories) and consume the remaining five days "normally." Between fasting days, allow one day.

- Alternate-Day Fasting Modified: Fasting every other day while eating on non-fasting days "normally." On a fasting day, you can eat 20-25% of your usual calorie consumption (about 500 calories).

- The 16/8 Method (also referred to as the "Lean gains method"): 16 hours a day fasting and eating all calories within an 8-hour window. It is recommended that women begin 14-hour fasts and gradually build up to 16 hours.

Whatever you choose, eating well during non-fasting times is still relevant. During the non-fasting times, if you consume many unhealthy, calorie-dense foods, you will not achieve the same weight loss and health benefits.

The right strategy at the end of the day is one that you can tolerate and maintain in the long term, which does not have any detrimental health effects.

Are you enjoying this book? I'd be extremely happy to hear your thoughts, so remember to leave me a short review on Amazon. It would mean a lot to me. Thank you!

Chapter 3

The Essential Tips for An Effective Fasting Diet

New meal schedule

Instead, she recommends starting slowly during the first week by, say, doing two to three days of IF and then "gradually increasing week to week." Taking things slow is not just a great tip for fasting, but a great tip for life (just saying '). Taking things slow is a great tip for life.

Having to eat and wanting to eat

Once you hear your stomach growl, you may feel like there's no way you can get more hours without food through X. Tune in to the cue for hunger. "Ask yourself whether the hunger is actual hunger or boredom," "If you are bored, distract yourself with another task."

If you feel hungry but not weak or dizzy, then sip a hot mint tea, as it is known that peppermint reduces appetite, or have water to help fill your stomach until your next meal, according to Savage.

During your eight-hour cycle, you need to add more nutrient- or calorie-dense foods or accept that this might not be the best plan for you. The addition of healthy fats such as almond butter, avocado,coconut and olive oils, as well as proteins, during eating times, will help keep you happy and full longer.

Eat when necessary

Technically, when following the 16:8 fasting method according to Hertz, extreme hunger and exhaustion do not occur. But if you feel lightheaded, listen up because the chances are that your body is trying to say something to you.

By definition, fasting includes eliminating some, if not all, food, so don't beat yourself up with small, and smart, to break your fast! -Bites, bites. Hey, your best bet? As Savage suggests, go for a protein-rich snack such as one to two hard-boiled eggs or a few slices of turkey breast (to help stay in a ketogenic (fat-burning) state). You should then go back to fasting, that is, if you feel up to it, of course.

Hydrate

Even when you fast, drinking water and bevvies such as coffee and tea are not only permitted but are encouraged per Hertz, particularly in the case of H_2O.

She suggests setting reminders throughout the day to lap up plenty of liquids, particularly during fasting times. According to both Hertz and Savage, aim to fill in at least 2, if not 3, liters a day.

Slowly break your fast

After going several hours without food, we would like to devour whatever is on the plate. But according to studies, chowing down in minutes is not necessarily beneficial for your body or your waistline. Instead of encouraging your digestive system to completely process the food, Savage explains, you want to chew well and eat slowly. This will also encourage you to have a clearer understanding of your fullness to prevent overeating.

Stop eating excessively

Just because you stopped fasting, on that note, doesn't mean that you can feast. You cannot only eat too much, it can leave you bloated and miserable, but it can also ruin the objectives of weight loss that probably led you in the first place to IF. To put it plainly, it's not necessarily how much is on your plate that will help you stay full longer, but what's on your plate. That takes me to the next tip for fasting...

Provide balanced meals

Ultimately, providing a hearty blend of protein, fiber, healthy fats, and carbs will help you shed those pounds and keep away from intense hunger while fasting. Per Savage, a good example? Grilled chicken with half a small sweet potato and sautéed spinach.

Hertz states that when it comes to fruits, you want to go for individuals with a low-glycemic index. A healthy blood-sugar level helps you resist cravings and is, therefore, necessary when it comes to falling pounds successfully.

Playing at various times

Although the 16:8 is often recommended by Hertz, she says to look at your overall lifestyle to see which fasting technique might suit you best.

For example, if you always wake up early, Hertz recommends eating during the earlier hours, like 10 a.m. At 6 p.m., and then fast until 10 a.m. the next morning.

Remember: The beauty of IF is that it suits you and your routine comfortably and flexibly.

According to Savage, another alternative is cutting yourself off earlier and eating breakfast later every day to gradually increase your fasting power. For instance, close the kitchen at 9 p.m., and then do not eat again until breakfast at 8 a.m. That's a natural fast of 11 hours! If needed, she says, slowly shifts certain times out.

Avoid fasting for 24 hours

If you aim to lose weight, it may be more helpful to consider your total caloric intake and focus on scaling down than toughing out a fast for a long time. Just take it from a study, which indicates that there are simply no further advantages than daily caloric restriction in fasting for 24 hours, Savage adds.

Customize your workout routine

First thing first: If you do a fasting diet, you can most certainly exercise. But you want to be conscious of what sorts of movements you are making, and when

It's important to note that if you don't, in Savage's terms, "adequately fuel your muscles," then you're at a higher risk of injury. So, on fasting mornings, you may want to try lower-impact exercises, such as yoga or steady-state cardio, and save the hard-core HIIT class for after you've eaten.

Keeping a progress notebook

Believe it or not, it will assist you with your fasting diet to maintain a food log. Journal of food for fasting! Yes, you heard that correctly. Although you might not chronicle as many foods, it will allow you to measure your progress by actively jotting down information such as any feelings and symptoms hunger level, fatigue, etc. that come up throughout Intermittent Fasting (IF).

It's crucial for symptoms such as dizziness, exhaustion, (unusual) irritability, headache, anxiety, and difficulty focusing, to keep an eye out at all times. Consider breaking your fast if you encounter any of these. And if you start feeling colder than usual, she says, that's even more of a warning to stop fasting. Be patient.

So don't freak out if you have a week or so of these (less serious) sensations. However, if these complications last longer and suffer symptoms such as the above dizziness, Savage advises that you dismiss the diet and try something else to help you achieve your goals. It's not worth getting sick for any amount of pounds-trust.

The Best Exercise Routine for Longevity

Here is the routine to optimize longevity that Longo recommends:

Walk fast every day for an hour

This need not happen all at once. For instance, if the train station is a 15-minute walk from your home, you do that every way you go, that's 30 minutes. Then you should select a coffee shop that is a 15-minute walk from your office and visit it every day. Those may not be your exact situations, but you get the concept of discovering walkable areas and going there every day. Walk everywhere, including faraway places on the weekend-do your best to leave your car all weekend long in the garage or driveway.

Practice 2.5 to 5 hours a week of aerobic exercise

Running, cycling or swimming are great choices, but it's not important what form of exercise you prefer. The trick is to work your body to the point of sweating and rapid breathing. Using a stationary bike and a road bike (go outdoors when the weather permits, otherwise ride indoors) is an easy way to meet this exercise threshold and make a point of cycling every other day for 30-40 minutes, and a total of 2 hours on the weekend.

To strengthen all muscles, use weight training or weight-free exercises to

This can be the classic workout routine, but when you take the stairs instead of the elevator, grow food in the garden instead of buying it, walk instead of driving, doing physical work around the house instead of hiring someone to do it, muscles also become stronger. Consume at least 30 grams of protein in a single meal within 1-2 hours to optimize muscle development while you participate in a tough weight training session.

Research reveals that much of the beneficial impacts are caused by the first 2.5 hours, in terms of how long you can exercise every week. A major Australian study of over 200,000 people aged 45-75, for instance, showed that those who exercised at least 2.5 hours per week at moderate to intense levels) had a 47 % reduction in overall mortality.

Going up to 5 hours a week contributed to a mortality reduction of 54 %. The chance of dying dropped by another 9% by ensuring at least some of the operation was in the vigorous category.

Another very large research involving more than 650,000 individuals in the U.S. and Europe found that mortality was decreased by 31% for individuals exercising at moderate intensity for at least 2.5 hours a week. The chance of dying was decreased by 37% by increasing the exercise total to 5 hours at moderate intensity (or 2.5 hours at intense levels).

Fast walking or slow jogging (faster than four mph), cycling (10–12 mph), or gardening are examples of moderate exercise. Climbing stairs or climbing, cycling (more than 12 mph), playing soccer, or jogging are physical exercise examples (faster than six mph). Therefore, there is definitely an additional benefit from up to 5 hours of exercise per week with some of it done intensively. But after 2.5 hours, there are declining returns, and by going far past the 5-hour limit per week, you want to stop overworking your body. Over-exercising can cause damage to your knees, hips, and joints over time.

My routine involves a casual run of 30 minutes in the morning, about five days per week. Thus, thanks to my morning run, I get 2.5 hours of moderate exercise per week. Then I add some vigorous exercise by playing squash for about 2 hours every week (I play twice a week, for an hour each time). In general, I'd say that I get about 4.5 total hours of workout per week.

And then I make a point of taking the stairs at all times. For instance, I take the stairs up to my floor from the parking garage at my office, a total of 111 steps. Every morning, climbing those stairs invigorates me for the workday ahead. Having meetings throughout the day on other floors allows me to rack up even more flights of stairs.

I walk whenever possible on the weekend. For example, take today's (I am writing this on a Sunday). This morning, I played squash for an hour and walked to the club and back for 15 minutes each way. I'm writing this from a coffee shop now, which is a 15-minute walk from my house. When I return home, in addition to my one-hour squash session, I will have walked for 1 hour. In a walkable environment, I place a high value on living!

In the field of strength training, my routine is the lightest. Every day, I do 145 pushups, but otherwise, I do not do any kind of weight training. Squash is a full-body exercise, but I would like to add some more upper-body strength training to ensure that my muscles remain strong as I age.

I considered exercise regularly to be an effective performance enhancer, and now I know how to exercise to improve a healthier lifespan.

Chapter 4
Intermittent Fasting Food List

The list of intermittent fasting foods should include:

1. Protein

0.8 grams of protein per kilogram of body weight is the Recommended Dietary Allowance (RDA) for protein. Depending on your health objectives and level of operation, your requirements can differ.

By reducing energy consumption, increasing satiety, and improving metabolism, protein helps you lose weight. Besides, increased protein consumption helps create muscle when paired with strength training. As muscle burns more calories than fat, having more muscle in the body naturally increases the metabolism. A recent study indicates that in healthy men, having more muscle in their legs will help reduce the development of belly fat.

The IF food list for protein includes:

- Pou
- ltry and fish
- Seafood
- Eggs
- Yogurt, milk, and cheese
- rains

- Beans and legumes
- Soy
- Seeds and nuts
- Whole g

2. Carbohydrates Needed

According to the Association of General Practitioners,45 to 65 percent of daily calories should come from carbohydrates. Carbs are the main source of your body's nutrition. The other two are fat and protein. Carbs come in different ways. Sugar, carbohydrate, and starch are the most notable among them.

Carbs for causing weight gain also get a poor rap. Not all carbohydrates, however, are produced equally and are not necessarily fattening. The type and amount of carbs you eat depends on whether or not you can gain weight. Make sure that foods high in fiber and starch but low in sugar are selected. A 2015 study indicates that consuming 30 grams of fiber every day will lead to weight loss, glucose levels improving, and blood pressure decreasing. It isn't an uphill struggle to get 30 grams of fiber from your diet. By consuming a basic egg sandwich, Mediterranean barley with chickpeas, peanut butter apple, and enchiladas with chicken and black peas, you will get them.

The IF food list for carbs includes:

- Sw
- eet potatoes
- Quinoa
- Oats
- Beetroots
- Brown rice
- Mangoes
- Apples
- Berries
- Bananas
- eeds

- Kidney beans
- Pears
- Carrots
- Broccoli
- Brussels sprouts
- Avocado
- Almonds
- Chickpeas
- Chia s

3. Fats

Fats should contribute 20 percent to 35 percent of your daily calories. Most significantly, saturated fat does not account for more than 10% of daily calories. Fats, depending on the form, may be good, poor, or simply in-between. Trans fats, for example, increase inflammation, decrease "good cholesterol levels, and increase "bad cholesterol levels. They are found in fruit and baked goods that are fried.

Saturated fats can raise the risk of heart disease. Expert views on this, however, vary. Eating them in moderation is wise. High levels of saturated fats are present in red meat, coconut oil, whole milk and baked goods. Monounsaturated and polyunsaturated fats provide healthy fats. These fats often, decrease blood pressure, reduce the risk of heart disease and decrease fat levels in the blood. The rich sources of these fats include olive oil, canola oil, peanut oil safflower oil, soybean oil and sunflower oil.

The IF food list for fats includes:

- Av
- ocados
- Cheese
- Nuts
- Whole eggs
- Dark chocolate
- ve oil (EVOO)
- Chia seeds
- Fatty fish
- Full-fat yogurt
- Extra virgin oli

4. To Have a Healthy Gut

Your intestine has billions of bacteria known as microbiota in its home.

These bacteria impair your gut health, digestion, and mental health. In many chronic disorders, they can also play a critical role.

The intermittent fasting food list for a healthy gut includes:

- All vegetables
- Kefir
- Fermented vegetables
- Kimchi
- Miso
- Sauerkraut
- Kombucha
- Tempeh

These foods will also help you lose weight, in addition to keeping your gut safe by:

- Reducing fat absorption from the gut.
- Increasing the excretion via stools of ingested fat.
- Reducing the consumption of calories.

5. For Your Hydration

The daily fluid requirement is:

- About 3.7 liters (15.5 cups) for men.
- About 2.7 liters (11.5 cups) for women.

Fluids include water, as well as water-containing foods and beverages.

During intermittent fasting, remaining hydrated is important for your health. Headaches, extreme tiredness and dizziness may be caused by dehydration. Dehydration can make these side effects of fasting worse or even more extreme if you are still dealing with them.

The intermittent fasting food list for hydration includes:

- Water
- Black coffee or tea
- Sparkling water
- Watermelon
- Cantaloupe
- Peaches
- Strawberries
- Oranges
- Lettuce
- Cucumber
- Skim milk
- Celery
- Plain yogurt
- Tomatoes

Interestingly, drinking a lot of water will help with weight loss as well. A study reviewed in 2016 reports that proper hydration will help you lose weight through:

1. Decreasing appetite or consumption of food.
2. Rising burning of fat.

For fats (75% of your daily calories)

- Nuts
- Cheese
- Avocados
- Whole eggs
- Dark chocolate
- Chia seeds
- Extra virgin olive oil (EVOO)
- Fatty fish
- Full-fat yogurt

For protein (20% of your daily calories)

- Eggs
- Poultry and fish
- Seafood
- Seeds and nuts
- Yogurt, milk, and cheese
- Soy
- Beans and legumes
- Whole grains

For carbs (5% of your daily calories)

- Beetroots
- Sweet potatoes
- Quinoa
- Brown rice
- Oats

The intermittent fasting food list for vegetarian includes:

For protein

- Seeds and nuts
- Yogurt, milk, and cheese
- Beans and legumes
- Whole grains
- Soy

For carbs

- Beetroots
- Sweet potatoes
- Quinoa
- Brown rice
- Bananas
- Oats
- Mangoes
- Apples
- Kidney beans
- Pears
- Berries
- Carrots
- Broccoli
- Brussels sprouts
- Avocado
- Almonds
- Chickpeas
- Chia seeds

For fats

- Nuts
- Cheese
- Avocados
- Chia seeds
- Full-fat yogurt
- Dark chocolate
- Extra virgin olive oil (EVOO)

Tips & Tricks on Getting Started with Intermittent Fasting for Women Over 50

Here are some tips and advice to get you started with Intermittent Fasting.

- **Stay hydrated**. Drink plenty of beverages that are free of calories, such as water, and herbal teas, during the day—avoiding a fascination with food. You must plan your fasting day around activities you enjoy, so you will not be thinking about food or obsessing over what you will eat next.
- **Resting & Relaxation**. On fasting days, do not do strenuous exercises, while light physical activities such as yoga, and walking around the house can be helpful.

- **Make each calorie count**. Now that you have chosen a plan for intermittent fasting, it is necessary to eat every calorie as nutrient-rich as possible. Select foods that are rich in fiber, good lean protein, and healthy fats. Nuts, Corn, lentils, poultry, pork, fish, and avocado are some examples.
- **Consuming high-volume products**. You must eat nutrient-packed high-volume foods, but for snacking, also look for low-calorie foods such as melons, grapes, vegetables with high water content, fruits or popcorn
- **Improve the flavor without the calories**. Generously season your meals with flavor-packed garlic, vegetables, sauces, spices and fresh herbs. These spices are low-calorie but rich in flavor and will help in feeling hunger less. Select foods that are nutrient-dense during fasting time.

Consuming diets that are rich in fiber, vitamins, minerals, and other nutrients tend to maintain blood sugar levels stable and avoid nutritional deficiencies. A healthy diet can also lead to weight reduction and good well-being. If you want to the 16:8 intermittent fasting, here are the tips that people find useful:

- Drinking herbal cinnamon tea throughout the fasting time because it can reduce the appetite
- Consuming water periodically during the day
- Watching minimal television to decrease sensitivity to food pictures that may stimulate a feeling of hunger
- Working out only before or during the feeding window, since exercise will contribute to hunger
- Try to eat thoughtful nutrition-packed food after breaking fast. Try meditation to encourage hunger pangs to pass throughout the fasting time.

Speak to your doctor if you're thinking about attempting intermittent fasting, particularly if you already have health problems such as heart conditions and diabetes. Expert advises trying to take it easy with the diet. The time window for feeding is shortened steadily over many months.

Also, as the specialist has advised, continue the medication routine. It doesn't interrupt the fast to take drugs and take the medication with calorie-free beverages like black coffee and water.

•*What if you require food with medicines?*

You may try to modify the fast in that case. It has been shown that overweight individuals can always do a lot of good even by taking medication with small portions of food. Simply work out a prescription with your practitioner that would support your well-being without losing the benefits.

You would like to ease into whether you are planning to attempt a fat fast or do intense intermittent fasting. If you are already consuming an unhealthy diet packed with quick snacks, fatty foods, and refined carbohydrates, you don't want to rush into these extreme fasts. One will find themselves in the bathroom for much of the day if one tries to rush into fasting. Instead, by first performing a 16:8 fast on its own and keeping off the junk food, build your way up to doing these intense ways of intermittent fasting. Some literature speaks of doing a fat fast over a few days up to several weeks at a time.

• *Your subconscious is the greatest barrier.*

It's really easy to follow this plan. You simply should not eat until you wake up. Then you have lunch and dinner, and then you go on with your day.

• *Weight loss is simple.*

If you consume less frequently, you will prefer to eat less in general. As a consequence, most people that pursue intermittent fasting wind-up losing weight. You might be preparing large meals, but in reality, consuming them regularly is tough. Keep monitoring what healthy foods make you feel better during fasting and keep cycling them. Intermittent fasting helps, but before a person incorporates carb cycling and calorie cycling, some people did not lose weight. By consuming a lot on the days, you exercise and eating less on the days you do not exercise, you cycle calories.

• *Prepare to get a lot of water to drink.*

For you, the safest lifestyle is the one that fits you.

Pay Attention to These Things When Starting Intermittent Fasting Over 50

You might find yourself grappling with hunger pangs as a fasting novice. Don't worry; once the body gets used to intermittent fasting, these are going to vanish. Ensure to drink enough water, particularly throughout the fasting window, during the day. Water can help keep headaches at ease, which will encourage you to stay feeling full. Tea, black coffee, and low-sodium bone broth are other drinks you can drink. Remember not to add milk or sugar to coffee and tea, or your fast won't do you any good.

Until you have achieved your fast, do not be pressured to overeat. Plan in advance: Load the plate with fresh, nutrient-packed foods full of high-quality lean proteins, fiber, and good fats instead of bingeing on anything in view. After the fast is over, these healthy meals will hold you sated and less inclined to overeat.

Here are some frequently thought-out questions for people over 50.

• **During the fast, can one drink liquids**? Yes. It is good to have water, tea, black coffee, and other non-caloric drinks. Do not add cream to coffee. There could be tiny quantities of milk or cream that are okay. They must be non-fattening. During a fast, coffee may be especially helpful, as it can curb hunger.

- **Is missing breakfast unhealthy**? No. The concern is that there are unsafe lifestyles for most traditional breakfast skippers. If you make sure that for the remainder of the day, you consume nutritious food, fasting is healthy.

- **When fasting, should one take supplements**? Yes. Bear in mind, though, that certain supplements can function best when taken with meals, such as fat-soluble vitamins, so look out for that.

- **Can an individual exercise while fasting**? Yes, easy workouts are okay. But remember not to overexert yourself. For women over 50, simple yoga, brisk walking around the house, and cleaning also count as a workout. Yeah, easy workouts are okay.

- **Would fasting trigger muscle loss**? All forms of weight reduction can induce muscle loss, so lifting weights and maintaining your protein consumption is crucial. One research found that intermittent fasting induces less loss of muscle than a daily restriction of calories.

- **Can The Metabolism Slow down during Fasting**? No. Studies indicate that short-term fasting improves metabolism. Lengthier fasts of three or more days, therefore, can suppress and disrupt metabolism.

Chapter 5
Intermittent fasting and Obesity

In the previous chapter, we tried to understand the reason for the failure of most weight loss measures and the mechanism of fat burning. The first and foremost requirement for fat burning in the body is the absence of insulin in the bloodstream.

Insulin is an important fat-storage hormone that our pancreas releases every time we consume calories. Frequent meals decrease the probability of fat burning in the body.

An Overview of the Historical Eating Patterns

Our eating patterns have changed drastically in the past few centuries. Historically speaking, gathering food was always difficult. We began as hunter-gatherers. Therefore, finding food was always difficult. Our ancestors never got food in abundance. They had to toil very hard to get food. It involved intense physical activity as well as luck. The odds of getting food were less. Getting one good meal a day was fortunate enough. This is a reason people may have died for several reasons but obesity wasn't among them.

Then, we shifted to agriculture. It increased the probability of getting food but still, the situation was nothing like the current era. Cultivating food was still a labor-intensive job and hence we were burning more calories in the process than we were consuming and hence the overall health of the general population remained robust.

The current age has brought great sophistication to food production technology. Getting food has become easy and less labor intensive. The food is also comparatively cheap and hence people can easily afford it. This has given rise to the abuse of food. We are not eating as per our needs but as per our desires.

Our body has evolved through millions of years in a food-starved environment. It likes to store energy. The mechanism is built in such a way that storing energy gives a sense of security. However, it is acting against our body as our intake has increased manifolds but the expenditure has gone down considerably. Labor-intensive jobs are carried out through machines and hence we have to rely more on exercises for burning calories.

This change in our eating patterns has led to problems that can only be resolved by addressing the underlying issues in food consumption patterns.

To burn fat there are some simple requirements:

- You must give your body the right conditions to facilitate fat burning
- You must consume less and burn more calories
- You have to make sure you check what you eat

If you can fulfill these three simple conditions, burning fat and maintaining the lost weight would become very easy and simple.

One Meal a Day is an easy way to fulfill all three conditions without going the extra mile in your daily life

Conditions Facilitating Fat Burning

As we have understood, fat burning is a complex process. The basic requirement of fat burning is that your body must not be in a fat-storage mode. This will not happen until there is a high presence of insulin in your blood.

When you begin practicing the One Meal a Day routine, frequent consumption of calories comes to a stop. One meal a day means that you will only supply the required calories to your body only once a day. Processing that meal and absorption of blood sugar would take another 8-12 hours. However, after this time, the insulin levels in your bloodstream would go down considerably as there will be no blood sugar spike. You will not be supplying more glucose to your body during this period.

This creates the required energy deficit. Your body has no other option than to begin using the energy reserves. The glucose stored in the cells lasts only for a few hours. Your body feels the need for energy and hence the liver starts metabolizing its glycogen stores. Fully replenished glycogen stores can last for 24 hours. However, when you start following the One Meal a Day routine your general calorie intake gets limited. There isn't excess energy to replenish the glycogen stores like before. Therefore, soon your glycogen stores wouldn't last even that long and hence your body would have no other option than to begin metabolization of the fat stores.

Consuming Less and Burning More

When you start following the One Meal a Day routine, your calorie consumption rate goes down. This routine generally doesn't restrict your calorie intake. However, as you can only have one meal in a day, consuming too many calories in a single meal always remains a challenge. Therefore, calorie control comes automatically. You don't need to count the calories anymore. You are always free to consume as much food as you can within a reasonable limit. You can treat yourself to the food of your choice as long as it is healthy.

Your calorie consumption goes down and your body begins burning more calories as the BMR remains the same.

Here, you can have doubt that wouldn't the BMR go down when the calorie intake is low.

The answer to that is NO.

When you begin dieting, you are consuming food at regular intervals but the calorie intake gets low. The body goes into survival mode as it is noticing a consistent reduction in calories. That doesn't happen when you are following One Meal a Day routine.

The single meal of your day will be providing calories in ample quantity and hence the body wouldn't feel the need to lower the BMR.

The times when your body needs more energy and it isn't getting any regular supply, there will be no insulin present in your blood. Therefore, your body would be in a position to start metabolization of the fat stores for making up for the energy deficit. Our body has an ample amount of fat to run the body for months without food. Running it for a few hours would not trigger any kind of survival mechanism.

Eating the Right Kind of Food

Food plays a very important role in our health. It also affects our eating habits and food cravings. If you are eating a carbohydrate-rich diet, it will load your system with instant calories. However, it would also create food cravings very fast. The same goes for sugar-rich foods. These things will make controlling hunger very difficult. Going without food for a very long period on such a diet would become very difficult for you.

On the other hand, if you start consuming a balanced diet with the right mix of fat, proteins, and carbs, it would become very easy for you to control your food cravings. A balanced diet also provides the required nutrients and gives your gut the right environment to facilitate good health.

One Meal a Day routine can help you in losing weight and burning fat. It helps your body in fighting the problems that have been created by frequent abuse of food that has been taking place for years.

It may sound difficult as staying on a simple meal for the whole day may sound like a very demanding thing. However, this book will explain in detail how you can follow this routine easily and it wouldn't sound as drastic as it feels.

It is important to understand that changing eating patterns is the only reliable way to manage weight and body fat effectively. It is a way your body knows very well. It would not only help you in losing weight and burning fat but would also help you in improving overall health biomarkers. You will feel healthier, rejuvenated, and full of energy.

Chapter 6
How One Meal a Day Help to Fat Burning

Until now, we have mostly discussed the issues prohibiting fat burning. We have also discussed the role of insulin in the whole fat-burning scenario. Before we move ahead to the next section and discuss the ways in which the One Meal a Day routine can bring a holistic change in your life, it is important that you also understand one major problem that is causing most of the health issues.

Insulin Resistance- Mother of All Problems

We know that insulin is an important hormone. We also know that it is the main hormone that facilitates the stabilization of blood sugar levels and the absorption of glucose by cells. But, do you know that your current eating habits are making your body insulin-resistant?

Insulin resistance is a problem that plagues most of us but we remain blissfully unaware of it. The reason is that it doesn't have any visible symptoms and it remains a chronic problem that keeps eroding your body. However, it is a problem that leads to most of the health issues we face in our day-to-day lives. Diabetes, hypertension, fatty liver disease, heart problems, fat accumulation, metabolic disorders, and many other such diseases are a direct consequence of this nasty condition that is caused by our erratic eating habits.

What is Insulin Resistance?

Insulin resistance is a situation in which cells stop responding actively to the signals of insulin and don't open up to receive glucose. This may not sound that scary but it is a bigger problem than most of the problems you may know.

High blood sugar levels are dangerous for your body. If your blood sugar levels start remaining consistently high then it can lead to the thickening of vessels in your vital organs. It can make them stiff and affect their functionality. That's why, as soon as your blood sugar level goes up, the pancreas in the body starts pumping insulin into your bloodstream so that the blood sugar levels can be managed fast.

Your cells also need a regular supply of glucose for maintaining their functionality. However, if their ability to bind with insulin goes down, they wouldn't be able to receive glucose and would starve. Therefore, insulin sensitivity must remain good.

How Does Insulin Resistance Develop?

Insulin resistance is a condition that develops when your cells start getting overexposed to insulin. It is like a nosy neighbor who is always sticking their nose in your doorway. One is always eager and welcoming to guests especially neighbors as long as they maintain a safe distance. But, imagine what if your neighbor starts banging on your door all the time and any time of the day or night?

This happens when you eat meals at short intervals. Whenever you consume a meal or any beverage that contains calories it gets processed and converted into glucose. This glucose mixes into your bloodstream and raises blood sugar levels. The pancreas senses the increase in blood sugar level and starts pumping insulin to stabilize the levels.

The insulin spreads across the body and knocks at the cells to enable them to receive the fresh glucose supply. However, if this process starts getting repeated very often, the cells start responding slowly to the insulin signals. This means that although your body would have a high presence of insulin yet your blood sugar levels would remain high and your cells would also remain energy starved. They stop responding to the insulin signals and they can't even absorb the glucose directly without insulin.

On the other hand, the pancreas would sense the high blood sugar level and would keep pumping more and more insulin to manage the blood sugar. This even increases the problem. The cells develop insulin resistance as they are usually overexposed to the insulin hormone. This increases the overexposure. The reception gets slower and slower and the blood sugar levels remain higher for longer than usual.

High insulin presence would also mean that your body would remain unable to burn any kind of fat and would constantly keep getting the signals to store fat. Therefore, all your weight loss efforts get washed down the drain if you have insulin resistance.

How Does One Meal a Day Help

One Meal a Day help in inducing the much-needed absence of insulin in your bloodstream. You can consume one meal in a day. This meal can be big or small as that would remain inconsequential in this respect. Let us suppose that you have your one meal of the day in the evening around 7.

Now, this meal would lead to glucose release and the pancreas would pump insulin. Normally, it takes 8-12 hours from your last meal for the insulin levels to go down in your bloodstream. This means that latest by 7 in the morning your body would have minimum levels of insulin. However, by this time, your blood sugar levels would be also low as you wouldn't be consuming a new meal anytime soon.

The cells in your body would get another 5-6 hours when there is no insulin banging at their door. This prolonged absence of insulin creates a favorable environment and the cells again start responding to the signals actively. This leads to the development of insulin sensitivity.

The greater the insulin sensitivity in your body, the better it would respond to weight management efforts. You would be able to lose weight fast and enjoy a healthier and fuller life.

Prolonged fasting is the only way to develop insulin sensitivity and lower the problem of insulin resistance in your body.

If your body is insulin sensitive, your pancreas wouldn't have to pump excessive insulin into your bloodstream, and hence the insulin levels would go down faster. This will also help in beginning the fat-burning mechanism faster.

Your body would come out of fat-storage mode faster every day and hence burning fat would get easier and would also get more time.

Therefore, if you want to begin fat burning, bringing down insulin resistance is a must.

Prolonged fasting is a good way to develop insulin sensitivity but that's not a practical way regularly. However, One Meal a Day is a practical method currently followed by millions of people to get the benefits of good health.

One Meal a Day also has loads of other health benefits besides fat burning that will be explained in the chapters to follow. They will help you in understanding the immense health benefits of following the routine.

Boosts HGH Production for Accelerated Fat Burning

The Human Growth Hormone (HGH) has amazing abilities. Our body produces this hormone in abundance and it literally builds our body. It aids in growth and helps in healing. If you want to build muscles fast this is the hormone to look up to. If you want to burn fat quickly, this hormone can help you like wonder. The importance of this hormone is such that bodybuilders and athletes started abusing synthetically produced HGH to a dangerous extent. It is a performance-enhancing hormone that can turn the tables for anyone. However, the use of synthetic HGH was banned soon.

Some of the Benefits of HGH

1. It accelerates the burning of fat
2. It helps in building muscles and promotes the maintenance of muscle mass
3. It also increases the stamina to do high-intensity exercises for longer
4. It boosts your immune system
5. It helps in the regulation of mood and also brings positivity
6. It has amazing anti-aging properties
7. It accelerates the healing, growth, and repair of damaged tissues
8. It increases your libido
9. It also helps in increasing the production of anabolic hormones in the body

The HGH Story

Our body produces HGH in large quantities in our growing up years as it helps in our growth. The production of HGH is very high in childhood and it reaches its peak in our teenage. However, as we cross our teens and enter into our 20's the production of HGH goes low. The reason is simple, we stop growing anymore, and hence our body stops feeling the need to produce HGH in large quantities. But, the production of HGH never stops completely. Our body can produce HGH if the conditions are right.

The Ideal Conditions for Production of HGH

1. When the production of hunger hormones is high in your body
2. When the presence of insulin is negligible in your body
3. When you are doing intense physical activity
4. When you are sleeping
5. When you face an injury or go through a trauma

Fasting is one of the best ways to make your body produce HGH in large quantities. It fulfills most of the conditions required for the production of HGH.

Our body produces HGH in high quantities when we are feeling hungry. Hunger bouts are common in fasting.

The insulin levels should be low to facilitate the production of HGH. When the body is in a fasting state, insulin levels go down.

When you do intense physical exercise in the fasted state, the production and effect of HGH increase. Therefore, exercising in the fasted state can be very helpful in increasing the production of HGH. It will not only facilitate faster fat burning but will also increase your stamina so that you can exercise for longer.

The American College of Cardiology states that fasting can give a 2000% boost to HGH production in men. In women, the production of HGH can rise up to 1300%.

So, if fat burning is your aim, HGH is the main hormone and you should focus more on increasing the production of this hormone. Fasting can help you in this direction a lot.

Muscle building is another forte of this hormone. It helps in the faster metabolization of fat and also facilitates muscle building. Your body will lose fat and build muscle at the same time. This is an advantage most people can never get through any other way.

Chapter 7
The Appetite Control

Our body has an amazing mechanism to regulate hunger and satiety. The system starts sending signals that you must stop eating when full. It also makes you eat when the stomach is empty. Everything has been perfectly timed and tuned.

However, obese people remain deprived of this automated system. They neither have any control over their satiety nor their hunger.

Let us talk about the satiety hormone first

Our body likes to store fat but this doesn't mean that it would want to keep hoarding unwanted fat too. Therefore, as soon as you start eating it begins releasing a hormone that signals your brain that the stores are being refilled. Soon when there is excess storage the hormones signal your body to stop eating. This condition is called satiety.

The hormone that signals this satiety is called 'Leptin'.

It is released by the fat stores. When you are unfed the release of leptin is the lowest. As soon as you start eating it increases and it is the maximum when you are full. The high amount of leptin in your blood would mean that you don't need to eat anymore.

Understand Why Most Obese People Can't Resist Food

Unfortunately, this system malfunctions in obese people and the cause of the malfunction are generally chronic inflammation in the fat cells. What happens afterward is the opposite.

When there is a chronic malfunction in your fat cells, they keep releasing the leptin hormone at a moderate level all the time. Leptin is released by fat cells and the number of fat cells is higher in obese people, their bodies keep releasing a high quantity of leptin hormone all the time. Whether you are in a fed state or on an empty stomach, there will always be the presence of leptin in your blood.

This should work as well because the presence of leptin would mean that you will feel satiated all the time and would eat less. This should happen in an ideal scenario but doesn't. High exposure to the leptin hormone makes the receptive organ resistant to the leptin signals. This means that even though your body is releasing leptin in large quantities, you may never feel fully satisfied.

Ever wondered why some obese people like to eat so much? They may not have hunger but they simply can't stop eating. It is not the temptation or love of food that causes the problem but leptin resistance.

This is a very serious problem as the body loses control over the fat-storage regulatory mechanism. Your body would keep releasing the leptin hormone at the same rate all the time. There would be no difference between the fed state and the fasting state. Higher consumption of calories would again mean more storage and hence there comes no relief from obesity.

Another major reason for the development of leptin resistance is the high presence of free fatty acids in the bloodstream. These are also released by the fat cells and the higher the amount of fat deposited in the body, the greater would be the release of free fatty acids. They impair the ability of the brain to register the presence of leptin and hence you never really feel full.

Fasting and a good diet can give you a break from this vicious cycle. When you begin fasting for longer periods, the incessant release of leptin slows down. Generally, when people eat at frequent intervals, the leptin release keeps getting stimulated. However, when your body remains fasted for longer than 20 hours, the leptin release also starts slowing down. Your brain can again experience the difference between the times when leptin release is high and the times when it is low and hence your satiety starts improving.

Inflammation of the fat cells is the root cause of the problem and that can also be tackled by eating anti-inflammatory foods. Food items rich in healthy fats and giving sugar, refined carbs, and unhealthy fats a miss is always very helpful.

Longer fasting and anti-inflammatory food can help in restoring leptin sensitivity in your body. You would experience better control over your appetite. You would start feeling full after eating which doesn't happen in the case of leptin resistance. In such cases, people simply keep eating but never feel full.

Chapter 8
Normalization of Ghrelin Release

Ghrelin is the hunger hormone in your body. This is a hormone that performs several crucial functions other than simply stimulating hunger. Ghrelin release promotes the production of HGH. It also helps in regulating insulin release besides promoting a healthy cardiovascular system.

Normalizing ghrelin levels can also help in improved cognitive function. People especially those battling with neurodegenerative disorders like Alzheimer's and Parkinson's disease can benefit a lot from normalized ghrelin levels.

Ghrelin release is highest when you are hungry and lowest when you are full. High ghrelin levels do promote HGH production but that only occurs when you are in a fasted state and insulin levels are low. If you are eating frequent meals and your ghrelin levels remain high, it can have adverse effects on your health. The high concentration of ghrelin in such cases will lead to overeating and you would accumulate more fat.

Foods with high added sugar content are bad for you. They do not suppress your ghrelin levels and keep getting added as fat. This increases the risk of obesity.

Intermittent fasting can help you in taking full advantage of normalized ghrelin levels. When you are observing extended periods of fasting your ghrelin levels increase and they facilitate the production of HGH. This hormone helps in burning fat and promotes muscle growth. The more exercise you do in the fasted state the better the results would be.

Longer periods of ghrelin release also promote cognitive function. You feel sharper and more alert.

Therefore, to get the best advantage of high ghrelin levels it is important to remain in the fasted state.

Your ghrelin levels are at their peak when you are hungry and go down after you have consumed your meals. Eating frequently and having foods rich in sugar cause cravings and do not lower ghrelin levels. You remain hungry and overeat as a result. This leads to obesity.

So, the ghrelin hormone acts as a double-edged sword. It can work to promote good health if you observe intermittent fasting but will lead to fat accumulation if you keep overeating.

Frequently eating food products rich in added sugar can also lead to adverse effects. Your ghrelin levels wouldn't go down even after eating and your hunger also wouldn't subside.

The ghrelin function is inverse to the leptin function. When your ghrelin levels go down your leptin release increases and you feel satisfied. However, if your ghrelin levels remain high, you wouldn't feel satisfied and keep feeling the urge to eat more. It will lead to weight gain.

Intermittent fasting can help you in avoiding this problem. It will normalize your ghrelin levels and let you have the complete advantage of high ghrelin release.

It is one of the reasons that exercise is always the best on an empty stomach. While you are a bit hungry your HGH production is high and you can exercise better and get the best fat-cutting advantages.

Chapter 9
Lowers the Risk of Chronic Inflammations

Most of the problems that occur in our body may look like the result of some particular incident but they aren't. All long-term disorders that our body develops are the result of chronic inflammation.

Inflammation in itself is not a particularly bad thing. In fact, it is the safety mechanism of your body to repair itself. However, the problem begins when the repair work starts once but never really ends. Such a condition is called chronic inflammation.

For instance, diabetes may look like a problem related to poor sugar control. One day you realize that your body is not able to manage the sugar levels properly anymore. For you, the problem began that day. However, the problem may have started years ago at least for your body. The tolerance level of our body is very high but everything has its limits.

Chronic inflammation of all kinds is bad. It can cause health issues like heart disease, hypertension, thyroid issues, obesity, chronic pain, diabetes, migraines, and even cancer. Not only this, autoimmune diseases like ulcerative colitis, rheumatoid arthritis, multiple sclerosis, and Crohn's disease are also caused by chronic inflammation.

- You may be at a higher risk of falling prey to chronic inflammation if:
- You are obese or overweight
- Your diet is unhealthy
- You don't do much physical activity
- You have too much stress in your life

Fasting for longer hours can help you in dealing with these problems. It brings down the oxidative stress in your body. Oxidative stress is a big reason for chronic inflammations to begin and spread.

49

It also lowers the presence of free fatty acids in your blood. The levels of LDL, triglycerides and bad cholesterol also go down in your body.

Fasting also helps in lowering the levels of C-reactive protein in your blood. A high presence of C-reactive protein increases the risk of inflammations.

These are the factors that cause chronic inflammations and fasting helps to lower the presence of all these factors.

Besides other things, the biggest victim of chronic inflammation is your brain. Chronic inflammation affects the levels of Brain-derived neurotrophic factor (BDNF). If the levels of BDNF are low, the neuroplasticity in the brain cells will go down. What this means is that your brain cells have an amazing ability to regenerate at a high pace, this power is called neuroplasticity. However, lower BDNF levels impair this ability and then cognitive functions start getting affected. Lower neuroplasticity can also lead to the shrinkage of the brain in size.

Fasting can help in increasing the levels of BDNF. Neuroplasticity also increases and your brain cells can regenerate at a normal rate.

Fasting also helps in curing chronic inflammations in other regions like your blood sugar levels, insulin resistance, fat accumulation, etc.

It is a great way to treat the problems concerning your liver diseases. Being the only organ in the body to have the regenerative ability, the liver is an amazing organ. It can treat most of the problems it faces. However, our current lifestyle and poor eating habits put a lot of stress on the liver. They can lead to inflammation and you may face problems like fatty liver disease. Fasting has a very remedial impact on this condition.

The best thing to counter inflammation fasting is that it lowers the oxidative stress in your body. Oxidative stress is the prime cause of most of the problems. When free radicals increase in the blood a lot, they cause oxidative stress. Fasting helps in the utilization of these free radicals for producing energy and hence the oxidative goes down.

So, if you want to stay healthy and fit, fasting can help you in a big way.

Chapter 10
Lowers the Risk of Heart Diseases

You can hear cholesterol in every other food commercial these days. The food production industry has brandished cholesterol as the main villain. However, it is not the whole truth.

Cholesterol is made from the fat in your body and it is essential for the production of various hormones, especially the ones required for making you virile and fertile. It has several other functions like it is used by your body as a Band-Aid. Whenever there is an injury to your heart vessels, cholesterol deposits are used to mend the damage.

The biggest heart problem people face is blockage of vessels and there are high cholesterol deposits. So, people conveniently blame cholesterol for the problem. If cholesterol deposits wouldn't have mended the damaged blood vessels, you may not have survived even this long. The real problem is caused by the Ischemic injuries your heart faces from time to time. Chronic inflammation, stressful life, and unhealthy foods are the primary cause of the problem and not the cholesterol.

Every time cholesterol mends the vessels, the arteries get narrow. Chronic inflammation even accelerates the process. If unchecked, this would cause atherosclerosis, a condition in which the cholesterol and fatty-rich plaque deposits restrict the blood vessels.

If you really want to lower the risk of heart diseases, it is important to root out the cause of the problem and that is chronic inflammation, stress, and poor food choice. Diabetes, high blood pressure, and a sedentary lifestyle also contribute hugely to the problem.

People even blame high levels of triglycerides for heart problems. Like cholesterol, they also have an indirect role to play in the problem. However, they are also not bad. Your body can use triglycerides for producing energy. The levels of triglycerides depend upon the kind of food you consume. Sugar-rich food would lead to higher production of triglycerides.

Fasting can help you in lowering your bad cholesterol and triglyceride levels. When your body goes into ketosis, it uses free fatty acids as the main fuel. The liver releases ketones that can metabolize the free fatty acids and triglycerides for producing energy and hence the risk of heart disease would be less.

However, it is important to note that high-cholesterol level is not the sole reason for heart disease and neither a true indicator of heart problems.

People have a great fear that if they eat high-fat food, they may face heart problems. This is not true. The reason for the high buildup of LDL or bad cholesterol in your body is insulin resistance and not high-fat food. In fact, almost 80% of cholesterol present in your body is produced in your liver itself. The percentage of dietary cholesterol is only 20% and it has no role in play in the health of your heart.

If you want to ensure good heart health, then your focus must be on lowering insulin resistance in your body and increasing physical activity. Fasting helps you in decreasing insulin resistance. If you also start doing exercise, the risk of heart problems would also go down. Exercises put your body under mind and positive stress. They also help in the release of nitric oxide. It makes your blood vessels expand a bit and hence their ability to absorb Ischemic injuries improves.

You can ensure better heart health with One Meal a Day fasting as it has a very high impact on insulin resistance. Your body becomes sensitive to insulin and hence the blood sugar levels in your body remain in control. If the blood sugar levels remain high for a long consistently, it will cause blood vessels hardening and this will go to increase the risk of damage.

Fasting also lowers the amount of visceral fat in your body. This is the harmful fat surrounding your vital organs. It dumps a lot of free fatty acids in the blood that cause inflammation. The lower the amount of visceral fat the better the heart health would be.

It is a proven fact that fasting has a very positive role in lowering blood pressure. Fasting decreases your salt intake and increases your water intake. As the insulin sensitivity in your body improves, the blood pressure also starts to go down. So, you will be less prone to heart damage from high blood pressure. Fasting is an easy and effective way to ensure good heart health. You can bring a big change in your health by simply showing some control over your eating habits.

Chapter 11

Helps in Diabetes

In the US alone, there are more than 110 million people who are either suffering from diabetes or prediabetes. Although no disease can be characterized as good this one, in particular, is the evilest one.

Diabetes makes you a slave of medicines. It is a disease for which medical science has no cure yet and all the doctors can do is manage the blood sugar levels to keep you running. Poor management of blood sugar levels can lead to severe complications and even multiple organ failures. High sugar levels also harden the arteries reducing the functionality of the vital organs.

Fasting is the only way to ease this problem a bit. It helps in the development of insulin sensitivity and your body can get better control over blood sugar management. However, if you are already suffering from diabetes, you must consult your doctor and undergo regular tests to ensure that there are no erratic changes in blood sugar levels.

Fasting can help you with diabetes in the following ways:

Helps in Decreasing Insulin Resistance

Insulin resistance is one of the major reasons for developing prediabetes which then matures into diabetes. If your body becomes more insulin sensitive, this problem can be avoided. Your body will be able to absorb blood sugar faster and there wouldn't be a problem with high blood sugar levels for longer periods. It also helps the pancreas by lowering the pressure on it to keep pumping insulin.

Helps in Weight Loss

Excess weight increases the problems of diabetes. You would be able to have much better control over diabetes if your weight remains under check. Fasting is a sure-shot method of bringing weight under control.

Gives a Boost to Metabolism

High metabolism plays a key role in managing diabetes successfully. Fasting is a good way to boost metabolism. Several studies have proven that you can give a great boost to your metabolism through fasting.

So, if you are suffering from diabetes, you must start practicing fasting. You must also keep your doctor in the loop as managing the blood sugar levels, in the beginning, can get tricky and the doctor might have to adjust your medications at regular intervals. However, it is a way through which you can bring a substantial change in your condition.

Chapter 12
Promotes Anti-Aging

Age has its effect on all of us and we age. As long as we are aging at the right speed things should be good. However, the current trend shows that people are showing signs of early aging. Stressful life, environmental factors, pollution, and chronic inflammations have a deep impact on our health. They make us age prematurely.

Most people consider premature aging to be a cosmetic problem. However, it simply isn't that. If your body is showing signs of aging it means that is something very wrong going on inside that needs your immediate attention.

There are 3 main factors responsible for early aging:

1. Oxidative Stress
2. High Free-Radical Damage
3. Low Glycosaminoglycans (GAG) levels

Free radicals and oxidative stress are interconnected as the higher the levels of free radicals are in your body; the higher oxidative stress would be. This would also cause chronic inflammations. We have already discussed that free radical damage can be reduced by the following fasting. It helps in lowering the levels of visceral fat in the body which is the main source of dumping free radicals. It also helps in reducing oxidative stress. Your body gets into a better position to fight chronic inflammations that may bring early signs of aging.

The main sign of early aging is brought by a slower rate of formation of collagen in the body. It is a structural protein found in the skin and connective tissues. GAG is the main chemical that keeps the collagen hydrated and your skin doesn't get wrinkles. It also repairs the damage caused to the collagen. The GAG levels go down in your body when the liver stops functioning properly. Fasting can help in reviving the production of GAG and you wouldn't have to face early signs of aging.

The chief hormone responsible for bringing this positive change is Insulin-Like Growth Factor Number 1 (IGF-1). If your body starts producing IGF-1 in healthy quantities, signs of aging can be reversed.

Some Important Ways to Boost the Production of IGF-1

Lower Insulin Levels

High insulin levels in the blood stop the production of IGF-1 in your liver. Your liver would only be able to produce IGF-1 if the insulin levels remain low. This can be made possible through fasting as we know that fasting has a very important role in keeping insulin levels under check.

Better Sleep and Cortisol Levels

The production of IGF-1 is higher when you are asleep. Because it is a repair hormone, its production is generally at its peak during your sleep. You can boost production by sleeping for optimum hours. The same goes for stress. The higher the levels of stress hormones in your blood the lower will be the production of other hormones as it puts the body in an energy conservation mode. Leading a healthy and positive lifestyle can boost the production of IGF-1 and lower the stress hormone.

Improve the Health of Your Liver

The liver is the place where the production of IGF-1 takes place. If your liver is healthy and functioning well it will be in a better position to produce IGF-1. Fasting has a very positive impact on the health of your liver. You can also improve the health of your liver by reducing the intake of toxins through healthy food. Lower intake of sugar and carbs also plays a very important role in the process.

High-Intensity Interval Training (HIIT)

HIIT has a great impact on increasing the level of HGH. The same goes for IGF-1. Its production also increases as during HIIT there is damage to the tissues and the body starts producing the repair hormone in large quantities.

Chapter 13
Autophagy

Autophagy is an amazing process. It is a marvel that our body has. It remained unknown to humankind for centuries and has been studied in detail in recent years. A Japanese scientist, Yoshinori Oshumi did a detailed study on the concept and found that our body has the inherent ability to treat most of its problems and the process through which it does that is known as Autophagy.

Most of the problems in the body are caused due to the accumulation of waste, toxins, and parasites. The body becomes inefficient in its functioning and several processes start self-harming. As long as the body remains in an energy surplus mode, it never feels the need to make the processes efficient as there is no need for the conservation of something that's present in abundance. However, as soon as there would be a severe energy deficit, the body would begin purging the inefficient process and that mechanism is known as autophagy.

Our body has trillions of cells and there are even a great number of germs that live inside our body. Some of these germs have a positive impact but many are simply parasites feeding on the energy produced by the body. Pathogens like fungi, molds, and bacteria come under this category.

When you begin fasting and your body senses that no energy supply is coming from outside, it feels the need to start autophagy. This process starts selective purging and roots out all the pathogens that are not playing any beneficial role in the body.

Our body produces millions of new cells every day. The process is unending and fast. In the process of producing new cells, some cells are not produced well. They have structural issues and they play no active part in the body. When the body goes into autophagy, it identifies all such cells and starts recycling them for producing new cells and also releases energy from them. This means that the body would start using up all the useless things in the body for producing energy. You will not only get new cells but the waste in the body would also get cleaned. These cells take up space and cause clutter. They may also cause problems in the body.

A part of the same process also involves stopping the growth of unwanted cells. Cancer is also a disease in which there is an uncontrolled and unregulated growth of some cells. When your body goes into autophagy it also identifies these cells and stops their growth. There are studies still going on in this direction but scientists believe that autophagy can play a very important role in stopping the growth of cancer in the body.

Treating cancer through other methods in a reliable way is very difficult as the cancer cells are also similar to your body cells. The medicines that kill cancer cells also kill normal cells. These cells behave in a normal way and have the regrowth also in the same way. The only difference between the cancer cells and normal cells is that the normal cells can function both on energy produced through glucose or fat whereas the cancer cells can only use the energy produced through glucose. When your body goes through autophagy the supply of glucose fuel stops completely. The ketosis begins and the cells start using the energy produced from fat as fuel. However, the cancer cells are unable to do that and they start shrinking.

Autophagy begins a catabolic process in which it starts purging all the cells in the body that are not playing an active role. It is a process through which the body becomes very energy efficient.

How to Begin Autophagy

Autophagy is an automatic process that would begin when you stop supplying energy from outside. It means that you would need to do fasting. Generally, it is believed that the body enters into autophagy after 36 hours of fasting as it starts feeling the need to conserve energy for the longer possibility of survival. However, once autophagy begins, even shorter fasts longer than 20 hours can give you the benefits of autophagy. Dr. Yoshinori Oshumi received the Nobel Peace prize in 2016 for his work on autophagy and further studies are underway to understand the benefits we can get from the process.

Autophagy has 2 main benefits:

Cleaning of the Body

This process starts purging anything and everything that's unwanted in the body. It is a very important process as it makes your body more efficient.

Stops the Progression of Diseases

Several useless processes are going on in the body like chronic inflammations that are not contributing anything and using up energy. Autophagy stops all such processes and brings you in a better position to fight diseases.

If done properly, you can lose a lot of weight through the process and also get healthier. Autophagy is a complete wellness concept in itself and can take you a long way toward good health.

Understanding One Meal A Day Routine

One Meal a Day routine as the name suggests simply involves eating once a day. It is a form of intermittent fasting. Therefore, to understand the One Meal a Day routine it is important for you to have a general overview of Intermittent Fasting.

Intermittent Fasting

Intermittent fasting is a very simple method of bringing variation in your eating patterns. It involves longer fasting windows and shorter eating windows within a day. It isn't complete fasting as you would be allowed to eat. However, it has a lot of health benefits as it helps in lowering the health risks and increasing your body's ability to lose weight faster and fight diseases better.

Several popular intermittent fasting routines are followed all over the world. The most commonly followed routine is 16:8. This routine involves observing a fasting window of 16 hours in a day and eating within the 8 hours window.

The next routine is the 20:4 routine or the warrior diet. It requires you to fast for 20 hours and have one or two meals within the 4-hour eating window.

Next comes, the One Meal a Day routine that involves fasting for 23 hours a day and eating a single meal within a one hours eating window.

There are other intermittent fasting routines like alternate day fasting routine that involves fasting for complete 24 hours and then eating normally the next day. This routine needs to be followed throughout the week.

There are also longer fasting routines involving fasting for longer periods up to 36 hours. These fasts can be observed once a month and they are very helpful in detoxification and cleansing of the body. They also help in kick-starting the process of autophagy.

Important Thing to Note

Intermittent fasting in general and the One Meal a Day routine, in particular, isn't a diet. The weight loss industry has engraved the idea of the diet with all efforts to lose weight. One Meal a Day is a routine. There are no elaborate rules to follow. There are no calories to count. There is no watch to be kept on what you can or can't eat. There will be no guilt conscious after every meal you have.

Intermittent fasting is a way of life. It is a lifestyle change that you will have to incorporate into your life. It isn't something that can happen overnight. You must incorporate this life change into your life slowly and give it the due time. The results will be phenomenal as the weight that goes away wouldn't come back. There will be no fear of weight relapse as your body would become capable of losing and maintaining that weight.

One Meal a Day Routine

There is no doubt that for anyone beginning intermittent fasting this routine can look scary and difficult. We have a very deep relationship with food. It is not only related to our physical needs but also has a psychological impact. However, if a person is facing a problem like obesity, then there is already an excess of stored energy that needs to be spent first. By showing some self-control and discipline one can easily follow this routine and get all the health benefits discussed earlier in the book.

Any kind of fasting requires self-control and discipline. To most people, 16:8 may look like a very easy routine. However, when you begin it, the process is equally difficult. You would need to train your body and mind to remain in the fasted state for that period. The same goes for one meal a day. It may look like a long and difficult routine but you don't have to begin with it. You must always begin with shorter routines and gradually move on to one meal a day and then it would be similar to all the other routines.

Hunger Is as Much Psychological Phenomenon as It Is Physiological

The biggest worry people have while beginning any kind of fasting is that they wouldn't be able to bear hunger. However, it is important to understand that hunger doesn't always indicate your body's need to eat. It is mostly your desire to have food that your body doesn't require. In fact, if you are battling weight issues, it means that your body has ample energy reserves to run the body efficiently. Going without food for a much longer period wouldn't harm you at all. Yet, the more weight you carry the more inclined you feel to eat.

This temptation of food is not a result of your body's need to eat but is caused by inflammation in the fat cells and food cravings. Both these issues can be handled easily by practicing fasting regularly and slowly increasing the fasting time.

Psychological hunger is usually very sudden and forces you to have food. The physiological hunger develops slowly and it gets regulated with time. The release of the ghrelin hormone that regulates hunger gets automatically timed as per your eating schedule. It means that if you are following a certain gap between meals, you are least likely to experience physical hunger before your scheduled eating time.

So, if you are concerned that you will not be able to remain in the fasted state for very long, your fears are unfounded. With a little practice and self-control, anyone can switch to a One Meal a Day routine and get all the health benefits.

One Meal a Day routine is very simple to follow and has the least complexities. You get one meal a day and, in that meal, you can eat up to your satisfaction.

There are four simple rules to follow:

1 Hour

You will get one hour a day to have your meal. This can be the most satisfying one hour of your day. You would have been in the fasted state for 23 hours and the hunger would be at its peak. Your gut would be ready to process the meal quickly as it would have easily processed your last meal by then. This is the best arrangement for your vital processes as well as your gut.

In this 1 hour, you can enjoy your meal up to your heart's content without worrying about the number of calories you are consuming. Remember, intermittent fasting routines lay great emphasis on 'when' rather than 'what' or 'how much'. This means that while having this meal you would have no guilt about having food despite being overweight.

1 Meal

You will only get one meal a day. This single meal of your day should provide you with all the nutrients, vitamins, and minerals. You will not be able to consume any other meal for the next 23 hours and therefore this meal should be very balanced and nutritious. You must choose the right kind of things in this meal that can provide you with the required nutrition.

The ideal ratio of the content of your meals should be:

- Fat: 70-75%
- Protein: 20-25%
- Carbohydrates: 5-10%

If your meal has this composition, you will be able to get all the nutrients without overstuffing yourself or feeling bloated.

The fat is compact and provides more calories as compared to protein and carbs.

The protein is also compact and helps you feel satisfied for longer without food.

You must consume fresh green leafy vegetables and whole grains to get your carbs. Green leafy vegetables are full of antioxidants, vitamins, and minerals. They also have a lot of fiber but add very few calories to your system. You can eat them as much as you want and they would keep your gut busy for longer. You must avoid refined carbs and sugar in your meals as they will not only cause cravings but will also load empty calories into your system. You would start feeling food cravings faster and the hunger would become unmanageable.

1 Plate

Keeping the quantity of food in mind is also very important. Eating after 23 hours can tempt you into thinking that eating more would help in remaining in the fasted state for longer. This is not correct. Overeating will only complicate things for you. If you eat too much you may feel bloated or overstuffed and that would cause discomfort. You must make it a rule to not eat more than one standard plate. It would obviously have more food than a regular meal but help you in preventing overeating. The better your balance of the macronutrients is the lesser would be the food on your plate. You should get around 1800 calories from this meal. This will ensure that your calorie intake remains in check and your body gets a chance to burn more.

1 Beverage

There are certain permitted beverages that you can consume even during your fasting period. Unsweetened black tea or coffee, fresh lime, and water are some of the things that wouldn't add calories to your system and hence you can have them in your fasting period too. However, in this eating window, you can have one beverage of your choice. It can be anything that you like but it is always wise not to consume beverages with very high sugar content.

If you can follow these four simple rules in your life, the One Meal a Day routine will have no complexities for you.

Preparation- Understanding the Difficult Part and Dealing with It

Weight loss measures of all kinds are difficult yet people follow them. However, we see that most people are never able to reap the full benefit of the measures. It is not the complete failure of the process or the practitioner but the difficulty of maintaining the routine that poses the real problem.

We all know that if we do rigorous exercise, we will burn calories. Our calorie expenditure will increase and if we can lower the intake there has to be some degree of fat burn. Yet, People with consistent gym memberships fail to get into shape. The same is the story of diets.

Diets are the most painful. They are restrictive and have a profound impact on the physique as well as the mind of the practitioner. Yet, you can see hundreds of people who have been on some kind of diet but haven't brought any significant change in their life.

People even take the extreme route of surgical intervention for weight loss. Bariatric surgeries are a norm these days. People get under the knife and have their guts altered surgically to bring a change in their diets. Procedures like gastric banding, gastric sleeve, or gastric bypass ensure that the body helps you in restricting your food intake. However, even the people who have been through these procedures experience weight relapse.

The most difficult part of weight loss is to follow a lifestyle that helps you in losing and maintain that weight. People generally give their complete attention to the regimen but pay very little attention to their lifestyle. They follow diets religiously irrespective of the severity of the routine. However, every diet comes with an end date. As soon as they get off the diet, they feel free to eat whatever they like and in whatever quantity they wish. Although they might have gotten off the diet, the body is always in fat-storage mode. Hence, weight relapse is even faster.

The same goes for fitness routines. People start with the toughest routines they can pick. They work very hard. They pump iron for hours in the gym and even start experiencing results. However, it is impractical for most of us to pump iron in gyms for hours regularly. Soon the reality kicks in that rigorous fitness routines are tough, excruciating, time taking, and exhausting. While we all want to lose weight, we also need to have our day jobs to run our livelihood. Soon, the realization draws upon people and the time devoted to fitness routines starts to go down. People even start skipping the gym. However, when people start the gym they also get on a specific diet to supplement their routine. Although they start reducing the time devoted to the gym, they pay little attention to the diet they had increased. The results are horrific.

The real problem is not that these weight loss measures don't work. The real problem is that they aren't lifelong options. It is very difficult to maintain difficult routines for very long. On the contrary, the body is always in fat-storage mode. It likes to store more and fatter as that is the best strategy from the survival point of view. This is the prime bone of contention.

Consistency in Weight Loss Strategy

If you want your weight loss strategy to work, consistency is the word for you. You can't pick one style for yourself and drop it at your convenience. Your weight loss strategy has to be a part of your lifestyle.

Slow and Steady Transition

Another problem with most weight loss strategies is that people begin with the most difficult routines as they want fast results. There has to be a difference between weight loss and instant noodles. The tummy tires didn't develop overnight. Trying to get rid of them instantly is a poor strategy. The results would be horrific and you would be sending shock signals to your body.

Imagine you had a pretty sedentary lifestyle and then one-day realization draws upon you that you are fat and you get on a rampage to shed the weight. From a sedentary lifestyle to pumping iron in the gym for one hour twice a day will be a complete shock for your body. The first reaction of your body would be a revolt. From muscle cramps and fatigue to dizziness, the symptoms can vary. However, one thing is for sure, your body is not going to appreciate it.

If you want any weight loss strategy to work for you, it has to be slow and steady so that your body can adjust to the positive change.

How to Incorporate 'One Meal A Day'

The best strategy is to go slow and steady as stated above. If you believe that staying hungry for a whole day would be a welcome change for your body, think again. It is neither correct nor advisable. There are several steps in-between that you will have to take. You will have to be consistent and move slowly.

Your body doesn't look at the food in the same way as you see it while you are on a diet. It is a reason diets are so much detested. You will have to get your body to develop the ability to stay without food. It can only be done systematically. Given below are the ways through which you can reach a One Meal A Day milestone with ease and stay on it comfortably. However, you need to understand that you won't get there tomorrow. It can take months at least before your body gets ready to remain without food for that long without food daily.

Every step of the way needs to be followed with consistency.

- You must stay at every level for a fortnight at least even after you have started feeling comfortable.
- You MUST NOT bypass any step.
- You must only move forward to the next step only when your body starts feeling fully adjusted to the routine.

First Step - Eliminate Snacks from Your Daily Routine

Snacks are the prime reasons our body is never really able to relax and constantly remains in the food processing mode. Snacks are highly responsible for the rising levels of insulin resistance. They keep your gut engaged and also confuse your system.

If you are overweight or obese, it means that you are in an energy surplus mode. However, snacks never really let your body rest. They are the prime reason behind blood sugar spikes in your body.

The first thing you must do is eliminate all kinds of snacks from your routine. This also includes all the sweetened beverages and tit-bits that may add calories to your system. You must limit yourself to 3 meals a day and believe me, even if they are unnecessary.

The best way to do this is to have a balanced diet. Any meal with a proper quantity of macronutrients like fat, protein, and carbs can help you in going from one meal to another without feeling the urge to have snacks.

The cravings that you may still feel are only a result of psychological hunger. Staying away from sugar, refined flour, and processed food that is highly laced with sugar and preservative will help you in doing so.

Try to eat food items that can keep your gut engaged for a long positively. Eating fiber-rich food items is a great way to do so. Such foods take a lot of time to get digested and hence you wouldn't feel unwanted food cravings.

You must adjust your body to this routine where you only have 3 meals a day at fixed intervals. You must learn to avoid all temptations of food in between your meals. Once you get used to this routine, follow it at least for a fortnight before moving ahead.

Second Step- Having All Your Meals within 12 hours

This one should be easy once you have eliminated snacks from your routine. It is very easy for us to remain in the fasted state for 8-10 hours. This is the time when we are sleeping. Make it a rule to eat anything a few hours after the sun comes up and have your last meal of the day before the sun goes down. This isn't very difficult once you have started exercising a little bit of self-control.

It can be difficult for you if your diet has a lot of sugar in it. A sugar or carbohydrate-rich diet loads your system with empty calories. While you are eating you start feeling fuller very fast as your system gets flooded with calories. However, this satiety wouldn't last long as although your bloodstream gets loaded with calories, your gut doesn't get much to digest. This confuses your body and the hunger pangs start developing very soon. That's why some people find it very difficult to keep their hands off the food. Such people start feeling hungry soon after dinner and may not find it unusual to raid the kitchen in the middle of the night.

The solution to this problem is also the right mix of macronutrients. The richer in fat and protein a diet you have, the longer you would be able to keep off your hunger pangs.

You must follow even this routine for at least a fortnight and only move ahead when you experience that the need to have food outside the eating window has gone away.

Third Step- Extend the Fasting Period to 16 Hours

This would be the beginning of the actual fat loss routine. 16 hours of fasting window can have a profound impact on your insulin resistance and it will help in developing insulin sensitivity.

Observing a fasting window of at least 16 hours a day will help your body experience positive stress. This is also very important for developing the ability to fight chronic illnesses.

Till this stage, nothing much would have changed. Only fasting hours increase from 12-16. You will still be able to enjoy 3 meals a day within the 8 hours eating window. There will not be any kind of food restrictions and you can freely eat anything you deem fit, as long as it is healthy. However, this is the time you must start observing restraint in your food choices and the number of meals consumed. Although you can have 3 meals a day, the 8-hour eating window doesn't leave enough room for distributing 3 meals if you are consuming a balanced diet.

You should ideally be having a heavy meal at the beginning of the day as you will be entering the active phase of your day. By the time you begin feeling the hunger pangs, you would be near the time for your last meal. If you experience hunger during the day, you must not have something very heavy as it would make you feel lethargic. Try to have some salad or fruit to suppress your hunger.

The last meal of the day should be comparatively light as you would not be working much as having something heavy can make you feel bloated or uncomfortable.

This way, you will be able to perfect the 16:8 intermittent fasting routine without experiencing any great difficulty. Having a balanced diet is critical as it will help you in going from one meal to another without feeling the need to have snacks.

16 hours can look like a long time to remain in a fasted state but in reality, it isn't much if you plan properly. The best way to carry it out is to have the last meal of the day as early as possible. Generally, the last phase of the fast is more difficult as the hunger pangs get intense. However, if you begin the fasting early in the evening, you can pass most of this time in your sleep. If you are a night person you can time your beginning of the fast a bit late as you would be getting up late in the morning.

In any case, you must have the last meal of the day at least 3-4 hours before going to bed. This facilitates proper digestion of food and hence the levels of insulin go down faster. It also helps in higher production of HGH which also aids your weight loss efforts. The load on your digestion system also goes down.

You should also start shifting the first meal of your day to later so that instead of having breakfast and lunch you can have brunch. This will again help in burning fat faster. The longer you remain in the fasted state the more your body would be bound to metabolize the fat in your body as it will not be getting energy from external sources.

Step Four- 20-Hour Fasting

Things start to get tough here and you should not move to this step until you have become very comfortable with the 16 hours of fasting. Once you can successfully shift your breakfast without any noticeable discomfort you will know that you are ready to move to the next step.

The 20-hour fasting is not very different from 16-hour fasting it only has the element of 4 extended hours of fasting. However, this may not be as easy as 16-hour fasting. This is difficult to master routine. You will most definitely experience hunger pangs as they are inevitable. However, the extended fasting hours and the hunger pangs aid the production of hormones that lead to fat burning.

At this stage, it will be very important for you to start consuming a highly balanced and nutritious diet. You get only 4 hours eating window within a day. You can spread a single meal within this four-hour eating window or have two meals, the choice will be yours.

The best strategy is to have something light like fruits and salads at the beginning of the fast and have a complete meal at the end. If you start with a heavy meal, you may not be able to eat much within four hours.

This is the routine you must follow the longest before moving on to the One Meal A Day routine.

Step Five- 23-Hour Fasting or One Meal A Day

Like all other fasting routines, this one is also similar to the previous ones in nature. You will need to remain in the fasted state for 23 hours and have a complete meal in the 1-hour eating window.

Hunger pangs will be severe and stronger and there is no getting around them. We have got so used to the routine of eating several meals a day that this routine may take much longer to perfect.

The only thing that can help you the most is a highly balanced diet. You must remember that most people with any kind of appetite will not be able to eat much in a single meal. Yet, you will have to consume 1500-1800 calories and get all the vitamins, minerals, and fiber from it. Proper distribution of the macronutrients is essential.

The fat content in your food must be 70-75%. You should include healthy fats like nuts, seeds, fish, cheese, eggs, etc. to get all the required fat.

Protein is required by the body and it must make up 20-25% of your food. Protein is slow to digest and helps you in feeling fuller for longer.

The ratio of carbs should be the least as they release energy quickly and make you crave food faster. However, carbs are also important as you get vitamins, minerals, antioxidants, phytonutrients, trace minerals, and fiber from them. You must include a lot of green leafy vegetables in your meal. You can eat as much as you want without counting calories as they add very few calories to your system. But they are full of other important nutrients. They also have a lot of fiber that will keep your gut engaged.

One Meal a Day routine is a lifestyle change that you will have to incorporate. This means that you must not take the liberties of cheat days. This routine doesn't prohibit eating or drinking anything during the eating window. Hence, there will not be a temptation to eat.

It is an ideal routine if you want to lose weight, burn fat, and stay healthy.

One Meal a Day may look like a rigorous and difficult-to-follow a routine but it isn't if you give your body the right conditioning and transition time. It is important to remember that obesity is a chronic problem. The fat accumulation in your body hasn't happened in a day and your body likes to accumulate fat. Dealing with that fat cannot be very quick. The quick weight loss methods are unreliable and the results are very inconsistent and temporary. The weight relapses faster than it went away and you would be standing back to square one in no time if you follow the quick fixes.

The best way to deal with the issue of obesity is to give your body the time to heal itself and counter the factors that lead to obesity. It is very important to understand that obesity is a result of the health issues your body has been facing, it isn't the cause. The causes of obesity are insulin resistance, diabetes, metabolic disorders, and other such problems. If you want to fight obesity then the fight has to be against all these issues and the problem would get resolved on its own. Once your body gets the right conditions, it will be able to burn the fat and utilize it for producing energy. You wouldn't need to undertake costly fad diets, overpriced gym memberships or medical help.

Sticking to the routine is the most important thing if you want to get rid of excess weight and burn fat to stay healthy and fit.

Chapter 14

Things to Expect

The Bad

There is no denying the fact that fasting for 23 hours a day isn't an easy task. There will be times in the beginning when you may start feeling frustrated. However, if you feel so there is no reason to be alarmed as it is common to feel so even on calorie-restrictive diets too. Symptoms of physical discomfort like headache, nausea, and weakness are also common. The good thing is that all these symptoms are temporary and would go away very soon. If you make the transition to 23-hour fasting slowly these symptoms may not arise at all while following the One Meal a Day routine. You would experience them early on and your body would get well adjusted to them by the time you get into the serious routine.

Still, some common symptoms may appear at several stages. This chapter will help you in understanding the problems you may face and the ways to deal with them easily. If you are experiencing these symptoms then there is no reason to worry, in fact, you should feel happy that your body has started to adjust to the routine and it would soon start burning fat.

Hunger Pangs

Hunger pangs are very common and even if you make the transition slowly as per the advice, you may still feel the hunger pangs troubling you. Hunger is a very important phenomenon. It is the push your body gives you to keep working towards bringing food. It is the motivation behind all the progress humankind has made throughout history. It is very natural for the gut to release ghrelin once the food in the gut gets digested. The hunger pangs are a signal to your brain to motivate you to eat. However, it is a mechanical process and every time you feel hungry doesn't mean that you necessarily need to eat.

Your gut releases ghrelin as per the schedule and it is mostly associated with the usual time of your eating. It means that if you are habitual of eating after you finish brushing your teeth in the morning, you will feel hungry irrespective of the fact that you ate a few hours ago. It is less about hunger and more about timing. However, the ghrelin release is always in spurts. It means, the gut would start releasing ghrelin at mealtime but would stop the release of the hormone after a while if you don't eat anything. It is a reason the hunger pangs are stronger for a while but subside later even if you don't eat anything.

The best way to avoid hunger pangs and the distress they cause is to keep yourself occupied. If you are sitting idle when you feel the hunger pangs the temptation to eat would get stronger. Your mind wouldn't stop thinking about food no matter how much you try. Keep yourself very busy in the last leg of your fasting schedule as the hunger pangs would be stronger and very real in this period.

Drinking non-caloric beverages like unsweetened black tea or coffee can also help in dealing with hunger pangs. These beverages suppress your hunger very much. You can also drink fresh lime water or plain water to push your hunger strongly. It will also help you in remaining hydrated.

Cravings

Cravings are nothing unusual. Most of us have cravings for food items, especially the ones that are sweet or spicy as mostly these things are loaded with calories and carbs. If your food has a lot of sugar, you will find dealing with cravings all the more difficult. The best way out is to stay away from refined sugar. The processed food that we get in the superstores is loaded with sugar. All the fat-free food heavily publicized in the market is also loaded with sugar as taking out fat from the food also takes away its taste. Hence, sugar is added to make it palatable. Reading the labels carefully before purchasing food items is very important. Food items that have sugar, fructose, and syrups as their prime ingredients must be avoided as they will cause cravings. The more you eat them, the higher will be the temptation to eat them often.

The same goes for food items with refined flour. Cookies, chips, cakes, candies, bagels, and all other such things are made up of refined flour and sugar. They have a negligible amount of fiber but are high in sugar and carb content. These things will load your system with empty calories but your gut wouldn't get much to process. Such things should also be avoided.

To avoid cravings, try to shift to fresh foods. Eat a lot of fresh fruits and vegetables. If you have a sweet tooth and you want something sweet, you can eat fruit. They have natural sugar that won't lead to cravings. The fruits also have a lot of dietary fiber that provides a lot of material for your gut to process. This is the healthiest alternative to harmful sweets.

You can only avoid cravings if you pick the right kind of food products. If you rely on processed food items then avoiding sugar may become difficult for you.

Headaches

When you begin any kind of fasting the most common side effect that you may feel is a headache. The main reason behind the headaches is the over-reliance of your body on instant sugar refills. When you are eating at frequent intervals, you are also dumping calories at regular intervals. It gets converted into glucose and your body loves to burn it. It is very easy to use fuel. However, when you start observing fasts, your body goes through ketosis and it adjusts itself to burn fat fuel. Fat fuel is comparatively difficult to burn but it provides a lot of energy. But your body doesn't like to make the switch easily. The headaches are the form of protest your body does.

The good thing is that these headaches are temporary and would go away as soon as your body makes the switch. Once the body starts burning fat for energy purposes, there would be no headaches as it would start getting the required energy effortlessly and without looking at you for it.

If you are feeling a headache due to sugar withdrawal symptoms, you can simply have unsweetened black tea or coffee. It will help in suppressing the headache.

Light-headedness

It is yet another problem that you may face in the initial stages of fasting. There is a very little chance that you keep experiencing it while you adapt yourself to One Meal a Day. It happens as your body notices a change in your eating process and it is battling between lowering the BMR and burning the fat fuel.

It is simply an indication of the fact that the ready supply of energy has ended and the body needs you to dump a few calories into the system. If you are feeling lightheaded after getting up or while walking, you must take precautions to avoid accidental falling.

This lightheadedness lasts a couple of days and your body gets adjusted to the fasting schedule.

Weakness

This shouldn't come as a surprise that you may feel a bit weak in the beginning. However, like all other symptoms, even this is not a permanent thing. While you observe longer fasting hours, your body feels energy deprived and hence there is a feeling of weakness. You shouldn't worry as it would go away as soon as your body starts burning the fat fuel. Our body can run for months without food on the body fat itself. One Meal a Day routine you will be eating 1500-1800 calories a day and hence there is no reason for you to feel weak.

In fact, obesity and associated disorders weaken the body's ability to absorb nutrients from the foods consumed. It means that you need to eat a lot more to get even small amounts of nutrients. Your digestive abilities go down. You start getting nutrient deficiencies and have to depend upon nutrient supplements.

Eating once a day helps your body and the digestive system in repairing or healing itself. The load on your digestive system goes down and it can absorb the nutrients from the food properly. You may also notice that you no longer require nutrient supplements to cure deficiencies.

Irritation

You may feel irritated at times and that is normal and happens very often when your body is looking for food. Irritation and mood swings are common symptoms. They are also sugar withdrawal symptoms and you don't need to worry about them. Staying away from sugar-rich food items and drinking permitted beverages like black tea or coffee can be of great help in treating the problem.

Frequent Urination

Whenever there will be a calorie deficit, the first thing your body would do is dump a lot of water. It would lead to frequent trips to the washroom. There is nothing to worry about this as it also leads to detoxification and cleansing of the body.

The important thing here is to remember to replenish the loss of fluids. You must drink water whenever thirsty. You must not stall thirst as that can lead to dehydration, headache, irritation, and other such symptoms.

Another important thing to keep in mind is that along with water, there will also be a loss of minerals from your body. This loss can be critical and hence you will have to keep replenishing the minerals. The best way to do that is to mix a pinch of sea salt in the glass of water that you drink. If you are suffering from hypertension, you must not mix salt without consulting your physician.

Heartburn, Constipation, and Bloating

Heartburn and bloating are common problems in fasting. When you get on any new fasting schedule your gut takes time to adjust. Meanwhile, it keeps releasing gastric juices at regular intervals that don't get any proper meal to digest. This can lead to a feeling of bloating. Heartburn is also part of the same process. Fortunately, this process is short as your gastric juice release system gets timed automatically very soon and you wouldn't have to face these problems for long.

Some people may also get constipated when getting on a fasting schedule. For them, eating a balanced and fiber-rich diet is the best solution. Such a diet would help in the proper processing of the food and would also ensure good health of the intestinal tract. This way, you can easily get rid of the problem of constipation.

The Good

One Meal a Day has a lot of benefits and most of the side effects that you experience in the beginning fade away. It has great positives in store for you.

High Energy

Once your body switches to fat fuel, you will start feeling a great rush of energy. The fat fuel is clean and produces a negligible amount of toxins and waste material in comparison to glucose fuel. Even a small amount of fat fuel will release a lot of energy. Soon, you would experience that you feel fresh and energetic.

No Lethargy

The most common feeling after having a meal is lethargy. We all like to sleep a little after having a heavy meal. It happens as the food loads your system with carbs and your blood glucose levels rise steeply. This doesn't happen when your body is burning fat fuel. It burns at a constant rate and there is minimal production of waste material and toxins. This also helps in avoiding the feeling of lethargy that people experience after meals.

You will always feel energetic and rejuvenated.

Positive Mood

Glucose fuel causes a lot of mood swings. When your system is loaded with glucose, you may experience joy, however, as soon as your blood glucose levels go down, you start feeling irritation, frustration, and panic. These mood swings can be very troublesome for many people as they are unable to explain the reasons behind their mood swings.

However, that doesn't happen when your body is burning fat fuel through ketosis. The fat fuel releases energy at a consistent rate and hence the probability of mood swings is very low.

Chapter 15
Setting Goals

Having a clear goal in mind is always very helpful. You can always judge whether you are making progress or not. When it comes to obesity, setting the right goal becomes all the more important as people have an innate fear of failure. Progress keeps them motivated and they can give a little extra if they feel they are making headway.

One Meal a Day is a tough routine. It requires a lot of motivation and nothing could motivate a person more than progress. However, setting the right goals is equally important. You must know the areas in which you want to make progress.

There are 3 major goals that people have when taking up the One Meal a Day routine:

1. Weight Loss
2. Maintenance of the Current Weight
3. Overall Improvement in Health Biomarkers

Weight Loss

If you have started the One Meal a Day routine for weight loss then you will be surprised to find that the success rates are high and the progress is evidently clear from the early stages. Yet, you must look in the right direction. There are two ways in which you can make progress.

1. Loss of Weight on Scale
2. Reduction in the Waistline

It comes as a surprise to many that although their waistline recedes while they follow the routine, they may not notice any significant change in their weight on the scale after a certain period.

Does this mean that they have stopped making progress?

The answer is no. They are making good progress but not understanding it clearly. One of the biggest benefits of intermittent fasting methods is that it not only helps you lose weight and burn fat, but it also helps in building muscles. The fat is voluminous and it makes you look bulky although it doesn't weigh much. The muscles are compact but heavy. So, while you are losing fat, you are also building new muscles. Therefore, the chances are that you may not lose much weight on the scale but there will be a significant reduction in the waistline.

Here, it is important to understand that weight is not the actual health problem whereas fat is a problem. So, if you are losing fat and gaining muscles you are making great progress.

You must take both things into account from the very first day. While you weigh yourself on the scale, you must also keep a meticulous record of your waistline to get the correct idea of your progress.

Maintenance of Current Weight

The biggest problem with obesity is that although you may be able to lose weight maintaining the same for a long is tough. This problem is noticed by everyone on any kind of weight loss program. People observe that weight relapse is a very common phenomenon.

One Meal a Day routine is a great program for maintaining your set weight. You will find that maintaining weight has never been easier. If you are following the set routine then the possibility of absurd weight gain is minimal. However, you must maintain a record to keep yourself well-informed and motivated.

Overall Improvement in Health Biomarkers

In the past few years, there has been a significant improvement in awareness about the dangers posed by a poor lifestyle, bad eating habits, and unhealthy food. It is a remarkable thing. Maintaining and improving health is even better than getting treatment for ailments.

One Meal a Day routine can help you immensely in that area. It is a routine that helps you in keeping blood sugar in check, improves insulin sensitivity, helps in lowering cholesterol, management of blood pressure and several other such issues. However, you can't track most of these things on your own. If you are following the routine for overall improvement in your health biomarkers then you must get a complete health checkup before beginning the routine.

You will also have to get the tests done at regular intervals to assess the progress.

You must mark all your accomplishments without fail as that would give you the push required to keep moving forward. Achieving milestones is the best way to remain motivated on a set path.

Chapter 16
Risk Factors and Viability of the Routine

All are not created equal in this world. What may be good for one, may not be the same for others. This qualifies for everything in life and even the One Meal a Day routine is not an exception. The routine is tough and has some risk factors for people falling under some specific categories. It is important that before beginning the routine you assess whether or not you fall under those categories.

Excellent for Weight Loss but Not So Good for Body Builders

One Meal a Day routine is restrictive. It limits your calorie intake and you may not get all the nutrients required for building muscles like a bodybuilder. If you are simply trying to lose or maintain weight this routine is ideal for you. However, if bodybuilding is your aim, this routine may leave you exasperated. Intermittent fasting routines are excellent for bodybuilding as they boost the production of HGH and adrenaline. Hence, stamina and muscle building get a great push. However, the One Meal a Day routine may fail to provide you with the kind of nutrition required for bodybuilding. You can consider other intermittent fasting routines that allow eating a bit more like the warrior fasting routine also known as 20:4 fasting.

People with Pre-existing Medical Conditions Need to Be Cautious

One Meal a Day routine is an excellent program to keep away problems like diabetes, hypertension, and heart problems. However, if you are already suffering from them, things may become a bit different for you. Pre-existing medical conditions put you at risk as you are already under the medication and leaving the medication for such long periods during the fast window can be risky. There is also a risk of blood sugar level fluctuation. If you have such pre-existing conditions then you may not get a level playing field.

In such cases, it is inadvisable for you to begin such fasting without proper medical supervision. You must consult your doctor and then only start the routine.

Pregnant or Lactating Women

The experts have a divided opinion about longer fasting for women. Although they agree on the point that fasting equally helps women as men, some experts believe that longer fasting can mess with the hormonal cycles of women. When it comes to pregnant and lactating women the experts think that they shouldn't fast. They have very high nutritional requirements as they are bearing the added responsibility of supporting another life.

People Suffering from Eating Disorders

If someone is suffering from eating disorders then also following the One Meal a Day routine is inadvisable. Such people are already under great stress and stretching it too far can create severe health issues for them.

If you are suffering from any health issue that requires long-term medication, you must not follow this routine without medical advice and supervision. One Meal a Day is a serious commitment and your body may not help you in the routine in such cases.

Chapter 17

Ways to Get the Most Out of The Intermittent Fasting Routine Part One

One Meal a Day is a great routine and it has immense health benefits. Anyone following the routine properly will get the benefits. However, you may still notice that some people make tremendous progress while others don't have such remarkable success. It is not the fault of the routine but the way they are living up to the routine that creates this difference.

If you want to have success in the routine you will have to understand the needs of your body. The body not only needs to lose weight but it also needs maintenance time. It needs rest as much as it needs exercise. Although fasting is good for you, the right kind of diet can bring a lot of difference in the results.

Given below are the four important things that you must give due attention to have success in your routine:

A Healthy Diet

Food is an essential requirement of the body. These days, food may have become the prime reason for most of our health problems, yet you can't run this body without food. The kind of food that you eat will always have a profound impact on your progress. We have already discussed that you need to have the right mix of macronutrients for a healthy body.

Fat, protein, and carbs all are equally important in set proportions. Yet, you must understand that every kind of fat is not good for your health.

Unsaturated fats can give a boost to your good health whereas saturated fats may increase the risk of heart disease. The worst is the deadly trans fats. You must make an informed decision while choosing the right kind of fat for yourself.

Protein is also important. While you must have the right mix of protein, relying solely on animal protein is not a very good strategy. Nuts and seeds also have high-quality protein. Eggs and dairy also have protein. You can also get good protein from legumes and pulses. Eating the right mix will help you more in staying on the healthy side and experiencing better results.

Carbs are usually portrayed as potential villains. All types of carbs are not bad. While refined carbs or simple carbs are bad as they can spike your blood sugar levels instantly, complex carbs are very different. Complex carbs are slow to digest and they don't spike your blood sugar levels. Additionally, there are several trace minerals that you can only get through carbs like whole grains, and hence avoiding carbs completely can be a very poor strategy.

However, you must always focus on having the right sources of these macronutrients in the ideal proportions to get the best health benefits.

Exercise

Exercise is essential to get the benefits of One Meal a Day. It is a way to force your body to burn those extra calories that would make the difference in your weight and obesity.

Some people may not be in a position to follow a strict exercise routine due to their weight and work routines. Yet, nothing can stop them from being active in their daily life. A sedentary lifestyle is among the prime reasons for obesity and you can't fight it by sitting idle or doing nothing extra.

The intensity of your exercise routine will determine the speed of your weight loss. However, those who aren't in a position to do intense exercises must do light exercises. Walking, jogging, swimming, yoga, and aerobic exercises are some of the routines that can be followed easily. Even if you have excess weight, walking every day is possible. Even if you have a traveling job and hitting the gym daily isn't possible for you, a few squats in your hotel room are easily possible.

One Meal a Day routine will create the right conditions to lose weight. You can capitalize on it by adding exercise to your daily routine. You must never ignore the exercise routine and should always involve some kind of exercise in your daily life.

High-intensity interval training (HIIT) is usually the best routine to lose weight. You need to perform some intense exercises in short intervals. This puts pressure on specific regions and has an excellent impact on your weight loss. You can perform HIIT on alternate days and do light exercises on resting days.

The important thing is to bring exercise into your life and increase its duration gradually.

Sleep

Sleep is equally important for your health if not more. It is the time your body needs for making a full recovery and doing the repair work. If you want good health, you can't ignore sleep. You must give yourself ample time to rest and recover.

The current lifestyle has become very hectic. There are deadlines, competition, worries, stress, and fear that have stolen our peaceful sleep time. Whatever was left of it was snatched away by social media and smartphones. The first thing that we try to look for in the morning is our smartphone. The last thing we have a look at before going to sleep is again the smartphone. It has the power to push your sleep aside for hours. It is eating our time yet there is nothing much we can do about it. However, to stay healthy and fit, you mustn't compromise on your sleep time.

It is during your sleep that most essential fat-burning hormones are produced. It is during your sleep time that your body can repair the damage incurred during the day.

One of the biggest side effects is also problems with sleeping. Sleep apnea is a reality known to most people facing obesity. However, mixing the right kind of diet and exercise can help you in getting good sleep.

Lifestyle

Our lifestyle also has a very important role to play in our health. Losing weight has a lot to do with a positive attitude. If your attitude is not positive, you may not get the desired results. Our lifestyles have become such that the scope of staying positive has gone down drastically.

We begin our days with a frown. We are always stressed about family, deadlines, competition, finance, the economy, politics, society, our neighbors and so on. The problem is that in most of these things we do not have direct control yet we are stressing ourselves with the tension and that is ruining our health.

We have stopped treating the day as day and night as night. We don't find it odd to sleep till late in the day or remain awake partying or watching TV till late at night. We are messing with the circadian rhythm of nature. This also puts a lot of strain on the body and contributes heavily to weight gain.

If you want to get the full benefits of the One Meal a Day routine you will have to ensure improvement in your lifestyle. It doesn't require much. You will simply need to give your body the required rest. Stop playing by hectic deadlines. Ensure that you maintain a reasonably active lifestyle and enjoy your life as much as you can.

Bringing positivity into your lifestyle can be very helpful in bringing down your weight. The more you feel crumbled down by weight the tougher it will get to get over it.

Chapter 18

Impact of Water and Juice Fasting on Weight Loss

There are several ways in which you can try to improve the results of your fasting. You can expand the benefits with water and juice fasting. The concept is as simple as it sounds. You will simply have to remove the meal and replace it with water or blends of fruits and vegetables.

Juice Fasting

It is a popular concept these days and people are following it in droves. You can simply blend the fruits and vegetables and drink them. Juicing them is not very advisable as it takes out all the fiber from them and you only get the juice which can spike your blood sugar levels. Juice fasting is something that you can do occasionally for 2-3 days. Doing it for longer than this might not have additional health benefits. However, you must also remember that you will have to remain extra careful while getting off your juice fast. 2-3 days of food deprivation calls for slow progression to solid food. This means that the next day you cannot begin with solid food. You will have to start with soups and then follow up with semi-solid food and eventually solid food. Not following this precaution can have an adverse health impact.

Juice fasting has become very popular as it is very easy to do and has good weight loss benefits. People are going after it with great enthusiasm.

There are some common reasons for doing so:

Fruits and Vegetables are Full of Antioxidants and Phytonutrients

It is a well-known fact that fruits and vegetables are full of antioxidants and phytonutrients. They help your body in fighting chronic inflammations. Fruits and vegetables are also high in vitamins and minerals and hence they help in providing extra nutrients and boosting overall health. Their anti-inflammatory properties help in boosting your immune system and you will start feeling more energetic.

They are Low in Calories

Fruits and vegetables are low in calories. You can bring your calorie intake to half by following a juice fast. So, if you want to follow a calorie-conscious routine for a few days you can do juice fasting.

They Help in the Detoxification of the Body

It is popularly believed that juices help in clearing out toxins from the body. Although studies have not been able to substantiate this fact.

They are good for Your Gut

It is a fact that juice fasting can help in improving your gut health. There are several healthy enzymes in fruits and vegetables that help in improving your digestive system. So, you can expect your digestion system to work more efficiently after this fasting.

Some Important Things to Note

Drinking juices in large quantities carry some risks. Certain juices contain oxalate which can cause the formation of kidney stones.

Too much juice can also cause diarrhea. This means that you will be at risk of losing too many nutrients and may experience weakness.

It can also cause an imbalance in electrolytes and you may start experiencing dehydration.

Water Fasting

Water fasting is a very common and safe way to fast. The biggest benefit of water fasting is that it helps kick-starting autophagy. This single benefit can outsmart any other benefit. When you are doing water fasting there is no intake of calories. Your body experiences a complete energy cut-off and it starts the process of running the body more efficiently to conserve energy for the longest periods. This means that it will become a chronic inflammation-fighting machine and a recycler.

You can do water fasting once a month for 2-3 days. Don't do water fasting longer than that as it may lower your metabolism. For the first few days, your body remains in an alert condition so that it can get food. However, when it doesn't get food for longer than 72 hours, the starvation mode kicks in. In this mode, the metabolic rate goes very low to conserve as much energy as possible and your body's main concern becomes survival. There will not be any significant weight loss in this stage and you may experience severe weakness.

Apart from Autophagy some of the benefits of water fasting are:

It Helps in Bringing Down Blood Pressure

Water fasting has a great impact on your blood pressure. People with high blood pressure experience a severe drop in their blood pressure. One of the main reasons behind this is the absence of salt intake during these fasts.

Lowers Oxidative Stress

Poor food choices and unhealthy lifestyles lead to a lot of oxidative stress on your body. This oxidative stress is responsible for causing several types of chronic inflammations. Too much accumulation of reactive oxygen species (ROS) takes place in your body. Water fasting helps in flushing out these ROS from your body.

Improves Leptin and Insulin Sensitivity

Insulin sensitivity will automatically improve when you keep the insulin release under check in your body. This happens on its own in water fasting as you will not be consuming anything with calories. The same goes for leptin. Your brain becomes more sensitive to this satiety hormone when you get off food for an extended period.

Although water fasting is good for your health, you must remember that getting off the water fasting is as important as the fast. Like juice fasting, you will not be able to eat solid food immediately after getting off the water fasting. You must start with liquids then move on to semi-solid food and finally eat solid food. This process helps your gut in adjusting to the change.

Understanding the Risk of overhydration

Someone who has been on a fast ever will surely understand the importance of water in fasting. Apart from the health benefits, it is the only thing that really helps in suppressing hunger pangs. You can fill your tummy with water and divert your attention from food for a bit longer.

The world praises water but no one talks about the risks of overhydration although it is equally dangerous as dehydration.

How Does Overhydration Occur?

Overhydration occurs when you start drinking more water than needed. Water is essential but your body doesn't like to keep anything that's not required. If you are drinking too much water then your body will have to pump it out in the form of urine and it would be an extra load. Besides that, when you are drinking more water, you will also have to pee a lot. Along with the water body also starts losing a lot of minerals too. It can cause electrolyte imbalance.

What is the Effect of overhydration?

The job of cleaning waste from the body is of the kidneys. So, if you start drinking a lot of water, it would put a lot of strain on them without reason. Overhydration occurs when you start drinking more water than your kidneys can process. This is not very healthy.

How to check for overhydration?

Keep a look at the color of your urine. If your urine is dark yellow, it means that you are dehydrated. However, when the color of the urine is like water it means you are drinking copious amounts of water and you must control your water intake.

How Much Water Should We Drink?

You should only drink when you feel thirsty. Don't drink water because others have told you or because you haven't had water for long. Drink it when you feel thirsty and you wouldn't have to worry about it. The water intake would naturally increase when you are doing some labor-intensive job like exercise or in summer. However, drinking water for the sake of it should be avoided.

When you begin fasting your water intake would increase as you wouldn't be eating anything and it helps in struggling with hunger but it shouldn't be used in excess.

One Meal a Day Routine on Keto Diet

Some people believe that all calories are the same. However, that's not true. When you eat a carbohydrate-rich diet, it releases a lot of glucose instantly but this energy is short-lived. Your body would start processing it fast as it needs to lower the blood sugar levels and you would start feeling hungry very soon. Fat and protein-rich diet, on the other hand, is very dense and releases energy very slowly. This is what helps you in going without food for longer. Fat and protein-rich diets are known as keto diets.

Now it is important to understand the process of ketosis as the reference would come time and again.

Ketosis

Ketosis is the process where your body begins to burn fat in place of carbohydrates. It is a very important process required for burning the fat in your body too.

Our body is an engine that runs on fuel like any other machine. It can run on two types of fuel, glucose fuel, and fat fuel. When you eat carbs, it releases a lot of glucose into your bloodstream. The insulin is dumped into the system by the pancreas to stabilize blood sugar levels. Insulin is a fat-storage hormone and hence until there is insulin in your blood, the body would never enter the fat-burning mode.

The ketogenic diet or keto diet is a fat and protein-rich diet and it has very little to no carbs. This means that your body stops getting glucose to burn for energy and hence it switches to fat burning. The fat is slow to digest and hence there is no energy spike and your body keeps functioning smoothly.

When there is no glucose supply from outside the body has no other option than to metabolize fat. The liver produces hormones that start breaking the fat cells.

How to Begin Ketosis?

There are three main ways to begin ketosis.

By Reducing Carb Intake

The Keto diets are rich in fat and proteins. They have very low carb content and the carbs are also complex carbs that are slow to break. This means that the body stops getting a ready supply of glucose and it has no other option than to burn fatty acids. The liver releases ketones that break the fatty acids and produces energy.

By Doing Intense Physical Exercise

When you do intense physical exercise, your body burns the glucose fuel aggressively and soon your glucose stores get low. Then it starts breaking glycogen stores and eventually there is no other option left other than using fatty acids for producing energy.

By Fasting

Fasting is also a good way to induce ketosis. The glucose lasts only for a few hours and the body has to begin using the glycogen stores for producing energy. However, if you remain in the fasted state for longer than 20 hours, the glycogen stores also don't last and the body has to begin burning fatty acids for energy.

One Meal a Day Routine on Keto Diet

One Meal a Day routine on a keto diet is a great way to push your body into ketosis. Your body already remains in a fasted state for a very long. The absence of carbs in your diet ensures that your body only gets fat and protein for burning. This is the same fuel as the fatty acids and hence remaining in a ketosis state gets easier for the body as it doesn't have to switch fuel types time and again.

If you want to lose weight, following a keto diet with the One Meal a Day routine will be the most helpful.

Chapter 19
Understanding Popular Myths

There are several myths regarding fasting and most of them don't have any scientific basis. You must understand them and the reasons not to worry about them.

Myth #1 Fasting Triggers Starvation Mode

This is a very popular myth for unknown reasons. I believe that people who have a phobia of staying hungry for a long have popularized this concept. The people who say this have no understanding of starvation mode and the way our body functions.

When you stay without food for an extended period, your body begins to sense the urgency of food. It knows that you need to be more alert and active to get food and hence your reflexes improve. Imagine starvation mode kicking on our ancestors. They would have perished away and we wouldn't have seen the light of day. Finding food was a challenge for them as they were facing extreme odds. The beasts they were trying to catch were much better than them in all respects. The animals they hunted were faster and had better powers of hearing and smell. They also had stronger and longer teeth and nails. If staying without food for a day could kick starvation mode, our ancestors might not have been able to get the next meal ever.

On the contrary, the body increases the reflexes after a few hours of fasting so that you can function better to get food. The starvation mode is a reality. However, it only kicks in after you have gone without food for around 90 hours. By this time the body starts conserving the energy to wait for the favorable times when you can get a resupply of energy.

Fasting is generally practiced for shorter durations and hence there is no danger of starvation mode kicking in.

Myth #2 Fasting Slows Down Your Metabolism

This is again a myth made popular by the food production industry which wants you to keep eating due to its vested interests. They believe that if we stop eating for a few hours our metabolism will slow down. We have a very robust metabolic system. It cannot slow down if you don't eat for a few hours.

If you follow calorie-restrictive diets, there is a danger of metabolism slowing down as the body starts noticing the lower intake of food. However, if you remain in a fasted state and you eat normally in the eating windows, no such change would get noticed as the body would be switching to fat burning to fulfill its energy needs. Studies have shown that during fasting periods, your metabolism increases by 14%.

Myth #3 Fasting Leads to Muscle Loss

People believe that if they don't eat food, the body will start cannibalizing itself and eat all the muscles. This myth has come into existence based on the knowledge that our body can use excess protein for producing energy.

It is true that if you eat excess protein than required your body breaks it down to produce energy. However, there is no truth behind the fact that it would start eating its own active muscles for producing energy.

On the contrary, studies have demonstrated that fasting leads to the production of hormones that help in building muscles.

Myth #4 Fasting Will Make You Feel Extremely Hungry All the Time

No, fasting will not make you feel extremely hungry all the time. Hunger pangs are a result of the release of a hunger hormone called ghrelin. Our gut releases this hormone periodically to indicate to the brain that food should be consumed. However, if you suppress your hunger for a bit long the ghrelin levels go down and you stop feeling hungry.

Your hunger pangs would also depend upon the kind of food you are consuming in your eating window. Consumption of a carb-rich diet will make you hungry fast as it gets processed quickly. However, the same is not true for fat and protein-rich diet as it takes much longer to process this dense diet.

Myth #5 Fasting Increases Stress Hormone Cortisol

Cortisol is the stress hormone that has several functions in our body. It is responsible for maintaining blood pressure, regulating the immune system, and breaking down proteins, glucose, and lipids. Cortisol levels in our body may increase on several occasions and that may not have any negative impact.

When you do aggressive physical activity, your body produces cortisol. It helps in the metabolization of fat for producing energy. It also increases your performance. Fasting also leads to a minor increase in cortisol levels but that only induces positive stress on your body. It doesn't have any negative impact.

If you are morbidly obese that would lead to the creation of extreme stress on the body and it would produce cortisol. In such conditions, it starts acting against your body as it senses the distress and stops the fat-burning activity.

Chapter 20

Getting the Best Out of Intermittent Fasting Routine

To get the best out of an intermittent fasting routine, you will need to follow the 4 golden rules

Proper Nutrition

Food plays a very important role in your health, and it also plays an equally important role in keeping you fit. Most people are attracted to intermittent fasting as they believe that it doesn't put any limits on food items. This is only one way to look at things. Intermittent fasting simply doesn't ask you to ban any specific type of food as that exercise only leads to a buildup of temptation and a negative attitude towards the process. However, you will have to maintain a routine in which your food will have to be in accordance with your health and weight loss goals. You can't simply keep dumping soda cans into your body and expect your weight to go down anytime soon.

Your weight loss would be proportional to the kind of food you have. If you take a high-fat low-carb diet, the ketosis process can begin fast, and you will lose fast. Whereas, if you stick to a normal sugar-rich diet, it may take very long for you to get results.

There is no doubt in the fact that intermittent fasting will help you even if you don't change your diet and stick to a carb-rich diet. The process will still help you in dealing with the issue of insulin resistance and all the other associated problems. However, burning fat would remain slow in this case.

You must only expect progress in the amount of effort you are ready to put into the process.

Healthy Exercise Routine

A healthy exercise routine is very important for faster weight loss. One of the biggest reasons for most health issues is the lack of ample physical activity. Our lives have got mechanized to a great extent. We have cars for traveling, and hence we don't need to walk. We have machines for harvesting, and hence producing food is also not a very labor-intensive job. We get readymade clothes. We can get pretty much everything done through machines. This makes most people into a couch potato. They start leading a sedentary life. Their energy expenditure goes down considerably. To lose fat and weight, you will have to work hard. A healthy exercise routine is the only way you are going to get that level of activity in your life.

If you are sincere about weight loss and health, you must develop a routine for exercise. There is nothing else that can help you in burning calories faster. Start slowly with easy exercise and keep increasing the time and level of your exercise slowly.

This way, you will be able to get better and faster benefits of intermittent fasting.

Optimum Sleep

Most people undermine the importance of rest and sleep in good health. You must give due importance to both these things. You must sleep for 7-8 hours every day. Our body does a lot of repair and maintenance work in sleep, and hence, proper sleep is vital. You must also not try to push your body harder beyond the physical limits. Giving the body the required rest is very important. You must take at least one day gap between High-Intensity Interval Training days. Doing HIIT without giving your body the required rest can make the recovery of the body difficult. A lot of muscles get damaged during exercise, which need time to regenerate. If you won't give them the time, your progress would always be slow and erratic.

Give your body the required rest. Do not push it beyond limits. Try to sleep as much as possible.

Maintain a Routine

Maintaining a healthy routine is very important. As I have been stressing from the very beginning of the book; if you are not able to follow a routine, this process of intermittent fasting wouldn't remain sustainable. The more often you break your routine, the harder it will get for your body to adjust to the change.

For instance, our gut releases a hormone called Ghrelin. The function of this hormone is to create hunger pangs and trigger the release of gastric juices. Our body releases this hormone as clockwork. If you are habitual in eating food at a particular time, your body will release the ghrelin hormone around that time only. This saves you from the troubles of unnecessary hunger pangs. However, if you maintain an erratic eating pattern, it would become very difficult for your body to judge the exact time to release the hormone.

If it releases the hormone early, you will have the excessive release of gastric juices and nothing to digest. This is something that leads to problems like belching and heartburn.

If it releases the hormone late, you may not feel hungry even at the time of having food. Maintaining a healthy routine is good for your body. It learns from everything you do and creates situations that are favorable for you. The lower the amount of variation, the less resistance your body would show.

Setting Milestones

Good health is an endless journey. As long as we are alive, good health should always remain our goal. However, when we start our journey toward good health, it is always important to set milestones to gauge our progress.

Milestones help in judging the progress, and also give us an idea for course correction.

Unlike other weight loss measures, intermittent fasting is not linear. It has a wide scope. People practice intermittent fasting for various objectives.

People follow intermittent fasting for 3 main purposes:

1. Losing Weight and Burning Fat
2. Maintaining the Current Weight
3. Holistic Health

You can be practicing intermittent fasting for any of these goals, but you can't judge the progress with the same scale. It is important that you set benchmarks for progress to ensure that the methods are working for you.

Your goals must also be in line with the kind of effort you are putting in. If you are putting in a lot of effort, and yet you are not getting the results, then you would need to do course correction.

Intermittent fasting to lose weight and burn fat

This is one of the most popular goals, as people these days are really struggling with weight issues.

There are two ways to judge progress in this area.

1. You should measure the target areas like the waistline, hips, and thighs with a measuring tape to see if the fat burning is taking place.
2. You should weigh yourself on the scale to see if the weight is going down.

There can be any one of the following scenarios:

- Your weight is going down, but your waistline remains the same

This happens in the first few weeks of beginning intermittent fasting. Your weight may drop drastically as the body starts dumping a lot of water. You must have patience as the body would start burning fat very soon.

- You are losing weight as well as your waistline is also going down

    This usually happens in the beginning phases, and your body loses weight as well as it burns fat too.

- Your waistline is going down, but your weight is not going down

This can happen when your body burns fat, but also starts building muscles. The muscles are compact and have more weight. Therefore, you may not see any significant change in your weight on the scale. However, this is a positive thing.

If your observation is something different, then you would need to revisit the whole process and determine the point where you are making a deviation or mistake.

Intermittent Fasting for Weight Maintenance

Maintenance of the existing weight is also a goal people have these days, and it is a very important thing. If the weight starts growing uncontrollably, the day is not far when you will be surrounded by a number of diseases. Therefore, you must get a weight bracket for yourself.

You can make changes in your diet and workout routines whenever you notice any significant change in your weight bracket or waistline.

Intermittent Fasting for Improving Overall Health

Improvement of overall health is a goal everyone must have. If you are healthy, the accumulation of fat is the last thing to happen. Your body is always capable of fighting all the excesses. To judge health improvement, you will need to take some tests before beginning intermittent fasting, and then keep repeating them at regular intervals.

Staying Motivated

Remaining motivated on the path of weight loss can be tough or challenging at times. Losing weight is a lonely road. People may praise you for the improvements you make, but no one is there to share your trials and tribulations. The pains and gains of the weight loss journey always stay with you.

Weight loss journeys can be really disappointing and painful at times. There may come times when you would want to put your guard down. There are points of disillusionment in the life of almost everyone passing through this journey where they start feeling the whole process is useless and worthless. It is not the journey that becomes worthless; it is our mind trying to find an excuse to get out of the tough situation. It is simply a reaction to a fight or flight response.

You must stay strong and motivated. These times are painful, but they pass away very quickly. You must draw inspiration from people around you, and take support from the people near and dear to you.

The best way to survive and thrive on this path is to find your support pillars. You can draw support from the following:

Friends and Family

This is the natural support base for everyone. It is a reliable support base you can look up to. You must confide in them as it gives you power. You can share your victories and failures with them, and hence, nothing keeps building inside you. You will always find yourself as light as a feather.

Sharing your problems or challenges with family and friends also helps in avoiding uncomfortable situations. If you are trying to avoid eating a certain type of food, the family members can avoid bringing or eating it in front of you. The atmosphere remains more empathetic.

Support Groups

You find people suffering from the same problems in support groups, and hence, you can relate to them and share your problems with them easily. Support groups play a great role in removing inhibitions. People don't feel strange, and they are better able to answer each other's questions. Most people have been through similar situations; hence, it is easier to find people with common struggles.

Professionals

You can also take the help of professionals like doctors, dieticians, and nutritionists. They are better equipped to answer your technical queries, and they can guide you in the right direction. If you are already suffering from any chronic illness, then you must seek the help of a professional; as regular monitoring of the problem is important for your very own safety.

Chapter 21

Intermittent Fasting Recipes

BREAKFAST

Trail Mix

Prep Time: 2 minutes

Servings: 6

INGREDIENTS:

- 1 cup sunflower seeds (raw)
- 1 cup almonds (raw)
- 1 cup raisins
- 1⁄4 cup flaked coconut
- 1⁄2 cup dried apricot
- 1/4 cup carob chips (optional) or 1⁄4 cup chocolate

DIRECTIONS:

1. Pour it all into a big container, cover it and shake it!
2. Store in a bag that is airtight. To preserve the properties of the essential fatty acids, place them in the fridge/freezer.

Roasted Vegetable Farro Salad

Prep Time: 1 hour 35 minutes

Servings: 4

INGREDIENTS:

- 1 tablespoon kosher salt or 1 tablespoon sea salt
- 1⁄2 medium-sized eggplant, peel on and large diced
- 1 cup cherry tomato washed and left whole
- 6 white button mushrooms, quartered
- 1 medium-sized zucchini, peel on and large diced
- 6 garlic cloves, peeled, trimmed and sliced
- 1⁄2 medium-sized red onion, peeled and cut into wedges

- 1 cup cracked farro
- 2 cups almond milk
- 1 tablespoon olive oil
- 1 teaspoon tbsp olive oil (15 mL)
- 1 tablespoon balsamic vinegar
- 3 sprigs fresh cilantro
- 1 tablespoon olive oil
- 1⁄2 teaspoon salt
- 1⁄2 teaspoon pepper

DIRECTIONS:

1. Preheat the oven to 200°C (400°F).
2. Salt the eggplant slices generously on all sides in a wide flat pan or baking sheet, toss to cover evenly, and keep for 30 minutes to release excess moisture and bitterness.
3. Drain the eggplant and rinse and toss it into a large mixing bowl. Tomatoes, zucchini, mushrooms, garlic and onions are added. Drizzle the vegetables with olive oil, season with pepper and salt and stir to coat. Move the vegetables to a pan lined with ovenproof tin foil. In the oven, roast the vegetables for 20 - 25 minutes or until tender, caramelized and forked. To avoid sticking to the plate, stir or flip the vegetables about 10 to 15 minutes into the roasting process. Set aside and remove the pan from the oven.
4. Meanwhile, rinse the ferro with water and drain over the sink in a colander. Into a 3-quart (3L) saucepot, add the farro and add in the Almond Breeze. Bring the liquid to a boil over medium-high heat to prevent boiling over then turn the heat down to a gentle simmer. Simmer the farro with the lid on the pot cocked to one side for 20 minutes to let out steam. Turn off the heat but leave the pot and close the lid on the stovetop. For another 5 minutes or until the farro is soft yet slightly chewy in the middle, steam in the pot. Using a fork to loosen the lid and the fluff.
5. Mix the cooked farro with the vegetables in a large serving dish and gently toss to mix until ready to assemble the dish. Whisk the balsamic vinegar along with the olive oil and drizzle over the farro salad. Toss to coat, and season to taste with salt and pepper. Add fresh cilantro and a squeeze of lemon to garnish. Serve it sweet.

Cajun Potato, Prawn
And Avocado Salad

Prep Time: 30 minutes

Servings: 2

INGREDIENTS:

- 1 tablespoon olive oil
- 300 g new potatoes (small baby or chats 10 ounces halved)
- 250 g king prawns (8 ounces, cooked and peeled)
- 2 spring onions (finely sliced)
- 1 garlic clove (minced)
- 2 teaspoons Cajun seasoning
- 1 cup alfalfa sprout
- 1 avocado (peeled, stoned and diced)
- Salt (to boil potatoes)

DIRECTIONS:

1. First cook the potatoes for 12 minutes in a pot of boiling salted water, or until tender, then drain well.
2. In a wok or a large nonstick frying pan/skillet, heat the oil.
3. Season with the prawns, garlic, spring onions and cajun, and fry for 2 to 3 minutes or until the prawns are hot.
4. Stir in the potatoes, then cook for an additional minute.
5. Transfer to dishes for serving and top with the avocado and sprouts of alfalfa and eat.

Baked Mahi

Prep Time: 40 minutes

Servings: 4

INGREDIENTS:

- 2 pounds mahi-mahi (4 fillets)
- ¼ teaspoon garlic salt
- 1 lemon, juiced
- 1 cup mayonnaise
- ¼ cup white onion, finely chopped
- ¼ teaspoon ground black pepper
- 1 tablespoon Breadcrumbs

DIRECTIONS:

1. Preheat the oven to 425°F.
2. Put it in a baking dish and rinse the fish. Squeeze the fish with lemon juice and sprinkle with garlic salt and pepper.
3. Combine the mayonnaise and the chopped onions and scatter them over the fish. Sprinkle with breadcrumbs and bake for 25 minutes at 425°F.

Sheet Pan Chicken And Brussels Sprouts

Prep Time: 40 minutes

Servings: 4

INGREDIENTS:

- 1 1/2 cup Brussels sprouts, halved
- 4 skin-on chicken thighs
- 4 carrots, cut on the bias
- 1 teaspoon herbs de Provence
- 3 tablespoons olive oil

DIRECTIONS:

1. Preheat the stove to 400°F.
2. Put the cut vegetables in a bowl and add 1 1/2 tablespoons of olive oil, 1/2 tablespoon of herbs, salt and pepper. Rub the vegetables all over.
3. On a sheet pan, place the veggies.
4. In the same bowl, add the chicken thighs. Drizzle with 1 1/2 tablespoons of olive oil, 1/2 tablespoon of herbs, salt and pepper. Rub the chicken all over.
5. Put the chicken in a pan.
6. Roast for 30-35 minutes or until you're done with the chicken.
7. Turn the oven over to broil and cook for a minute or two if you prefer a crispier vegetable or chicken skin. Carefully watch, or it'll burn.

Cauliflower Pizza Crust

Prep Time: 1 hour 10 minutes

Servings: 4

INGREDIENTS:

- 1 egg, beaten
- 4 cups raw cauliflower, rice or 1 medium cauliflower head
- 1 cup chevre cheese or 1 cup other soft cheese
- 1 pinch salt
- 1 teaspoon dried oregano

DIRECTIONS:

1. Preheat to 400°F in your oven.
2. Place the still-uncooked cauliflower florets in a food processor and mix until a rice-like consistency is achieved.
3. Fill a big pot and bring it to a boil with around an inch of water. Connect the "rice" and cover; cook for 5 minutes or so. Drain the strainer into a fine-mesh one.
4. THIS IS THE SECRET: Move it to a clean, thin dishtowel once you've strained the rice. In the dishtowel, cover the steamed rice, curl it and suck out all the excess moisture! It's amazing how much extra liquid will be released, leaving you with a good dry crust of the pizza.
5. Mix your strained rice, beaten egg, goat's cheese, and spices in a big bowl. (Don't fear using your hands! You want it mixed well.) It's not going to be like every pizza dough you've ever dealt with, yet don't worry, it's going to stay together!
6. On a baking sheet lined with parchment paper, press the dough out. Keep the dough about 3/8" thick, and make the edges a little higher for a "crust" effect, if you like. (It must be lined with parchment paper, or it will stick.)"
7. Bake at 400°F for 35-40 minutes. The crust should be firm and when done, golden brown.
8. Now's the time to add sauce, cheese, and any other toppings you want to all your favorites. Put the pizza back in the oven for 400F and bake for an additional 5-10 minutes, only until the cheese is hot and bubbly.
9. Cut and quickly serve!

Sweet Potato And Black Bean Burrito

Prep Time: 1 hour 5 minutes

Yield: 8-12 portions

INGREDIENTS:

- 5 cups peeled cubed sweet potatoes
- 2 teaspoons other vegetable oil or two teaspoons broth
- 1/2 teaspoon salt
- 3 1/2 cups diced onions
- 1 tablespoon minced fresh green chili pepper
- 4 garlic cloves, minced (or pressed)
- 4 teaspoons ground cumin
- 4 1/2 cups cooked black beans
- 4 teaspoons ground coriander
- 2/3 cup lightly packed cilantro leaf
- 1 teaspoon salt
- 12 (10 inches) flour tortillas
- 2 tablespoons fresh lemon juice
- Fresh salsa

DIRECTIONS:

1. Preheat the oven to 350°F.
2. Place the salt and water in a medium saucepan to cover the sweet potatoes.
3. Cover and bring to a boil, then simmer for about 10 minutes, until tender.
4. Drain yourself and set aside.
5. Heat the oil in a medium saucepan or skillet while the sweet potatoes are frying, and add the onions, garlic, and chili.
6. On medium-low heat, cover and cook, occasionally stirring, until the onions are tender, around 7 minutes.
7. Add cumin and coriander and cook, constantly stirring, for 2 to 3 minutes longer.
8. Remove and set aside from the sun.
9. Combine the black beans, lemon juice, cilantro, salt and cooked sweet potatoes in a food processor and puree.
10. In a large mixing bowl, pass the sweet potato mixture and blend in the cooked onions and spices.
11. Oil a large baking dish lightly.
12. In the center of each tortilla, pour about 2/3 cup of filling; Now roll it up and place it in the baking dish, seam side down.
13. Cover thoroughly with foil and bake for 30 minutes or so, until sweet.
14. Serve with salsa topping.

Slow Cooker Black Eyed Peas

Prep Time: 10 hours 5 minutes

Servings: 6

INGREDIENTS:
- 1 small ham hock
- 1 (16 ounces) bag dried black-eyed peas
- 1 (14 1/2 ounces) can diced tomatoes with green chilies
- 1 (14 1/2 ounces) can Del Monte zesty jalapeno pepper diced tomato
- 1 stalk celery, chopped
- 2 (10 1/2 ounces) cans chicken broth

DIRECTIONS:
1. Following the directions on the bag, pre-soak black-eyed peas.
2. Combine all ingredients and cook for 9-10 hours on low heat.

Peach Berry Smoothie

Prep Time: 5 minutes

Servings: 1

INGREDIENTS:
- 1 cup frozen peaches
- 1/2 cup Greek yogurt
- 1/4 cup coconut milk
- 1/2 teaspoon almond flavoring

DIRECTIONS:
1. In a high-speed blender, blend the peaches with almond flavoring.
2. Check and change the thickness accordingly. For thinner, add more milk and for thicker, more peaches.
3. Gorgeous toppings such as chia seeds, berries and slivered almonds are on top. Enjoy.

Sweet Potato Curry With Spinach

Prep Time: 30 minutes

Servings: 6

INGREDIENTS:

- 1 -2 teaspoon canola oil
- 1 tablespoon cumin
- 2 tablespoons curry powder
- 1 teaspoon cinnamon
- 1⁄2 large sweet onions, chopped or two scallions, thinly sliced
- 10 ounces fresh spinach washed
- 1 (14 1/2 ounces) can chickpeas, rinsed and drained
- 2 large sweet potatoes, peeled and diced (about 2 pounds)
- 1⁄2 cup water
- 1⁄4 cup chopped cilantro
- 1 can diced tomatoes
- Basmati rice or brown rice, for serving

DIRECTIONS:

1. Whatever you like, you can choose to cook sweet potatoes.
2. I enjoy peeling, slicing and steaming mine for about 15 minutes in a veggie steamer.
3. Fit well baking or boiling, too.
4. Heat 2 tsp of vegetable oil while the sweet potatoes are cooking.
5. Add the onions and sauté for 2-3 minutes, or until tender.
6. Add the curry powder, cumin, and cinnamon, then stir to cover the onions with the spices evenly.
7. Stir in the tomatoes and their juices, and stir in the chickpeas to blend.
8. Add half a cup of water and lift the heat for about a minute or two to a high simmer.
9. Then add fresh spinach, stirring to cover with cooking liquid, a few handfuls at a time.
10. Cover and boil until just wilted, about 3 minutes, when all the spinach is added to the pan.
11. Apply to the liquid the cooked sweet potatoes, and stir to coat.
12. Simmer for another 3-5 minutes, or until you mix the flavors well.
13. Move to a dish for serving, toss with fresh cilantro and serve sweet.
14. This dish is served beautifully over basmati or brown rice.

Poached Eggs And Avocado Toasts

Prep Time: 15 minutes

Servings: 4

INGREDIENTS:

- 2 ripe avocados
- 4 eggs
- 2 teaspoons lemon juice
- 1 cup cheese
- 4 slices thick bread
- 4 teaspoons butter
- Salt and freshly ground black pepper

DIRECTIONS:

1. Using your favorite technique, poach eggs.
2. Meanwhile, the avocados are cut in half, and the stones are removed.
3. Scoop out the flesh in a bowl with a spoon and apply the lemon or lime juice and salt & pepper.
4. Mash using a fork.
5. Bread toast and spread with butter.
6. On each slice of buttered toast, spread the avocado mix and top each one with a poached egg.
7. Sprinkle the grated cheese over it and serve immediately.
8. These are also good with tomato halves on the side, either fresh or grilled.

French Vanilla Almond Granola

Prep Time: 2 hours 10 minutes

Servings: 12

Yield: 12 ½ cups

INGREDIENTS:
- ½ cup sliced almonds
- 3 ½ cups old-fashioned oats
- ½ cup water
- ¼ teaspoon salt
- ½ cup natural cane sugar
- 1 tablespoon vanilla extract
- 1/4 cup grapeseed oil

DIRECTIONS:
1. Heat the oven to 200°F. Use parchment paper to line a big, rimmed cookie sheet.
2. Combine the oats and the almonds in a large dish.
3. Mix the sugar and salt into the water in a small saucepan over medium heat. Stir and cook until the sugar has dissolved. Withdraw from the sun. Stir in the vanilla and canola oil. Pour the oat and almond mixture into the mixture and stir until well mixed.
4. On the lined cookie sheet, spread the mixture out and bake for 2 hours, or until tender to the touch. Oh, don't stir! Remove from the oven and allow to cool into chunks before breaking apart. Store in a bag that is air-tight.

Millet And Quinoa Mediterranean Salad

Prep Time: 40 minutes

Servings: 3-4

Yield: 5 cups

INGREDIENTS:

- 1 cup water
- ½ cup millet
- ¾ cup water
- 1 English cucumber, diced
- ½ cup quinoa (red, white, or black)
- 1 sweet pepper, seeded, diced
- 1 tomato, ripe, seeds squeezed out, diced
- ½ red onion, sliced thin
- 200 g feta cheese, diced
- 1 (10 ounces) can make large white beans, drained
- 1 garlic clove, pressed
- ¼ teaspoon cayenne pepper
- ¼ cup pine nuts
- 1 lemon, juice of
- 2 teaspoons dried dill
- 1 tablespoon olive oil
- Fresh ground pepper, to taste

DIRECTIONS:

1. Bring 1 cup of water and 1 millet to a boil, reduce heat and simmer for 5 minutes; turn off the heat and let sit for 15 minutes.
2. Bring to a boil quinoa and 3/4 cup water, reduce heat, and simmer, covered, for 12-14 minutes; fluff.
3. Combine and toss all ingredients; chill. Enjoy!

Grilled Lemon Salmon

Prep Time: 27 minutes

Servings: 4

INGREDIENTS:

- ½ teaspoon pepper
- ½ teaspoon salt
- 2 teaspoons fresh dill
- ½ teaspoon garlic powder
- ¼ cup packed brown sugar
- 1 chicken bouillon cube, mixed with
- 1 ½ pound salmon fillets
- 3 tablespoons oil
- 3 tablespoons soy sauce
- 3 tablespoons water
- 1 lemon, thinly sliced
- 2 slices onions, separated into rings
- 4 tablespoons finely chopped green onions

DIRECTIONS:

1. Sprinkle some salmon with dill, pepper, salt and garlic powder.
2. Place them in a shallow pan of glass.
3. Mix the sugar, the chicken bouillon, the oil, the soy sauce and the green onions. Pour the salmon over.
4. Cover and refrigerate for 1 hour, turning once.
5. Drain the marinade and dump it.
6. Put the lemon and onion on the grill over medium heat and place on top.
7. Cover and cook for 20 minutes or until you're finished with the fish.

Avocado Quesadillas

Prep Time: 31minutes

Servings: 2

INGREDIENTS:

- 1 ripe avocado, peeled and pitted
- 2 teaspoons fresh lemon juice
- 1⁄4 teaspoon Tabasco sauce
- 1⁄2 teaspoon vegetable oil
- 1 tablespoon chopped red onion
- Salt and pepper
- 3 tablespoons chopped fresh coriander
- 1⁄4 cup sour cream
- 24 inches flour tortillas
- 1⁄3 cup shredded cheese
- 2 vine-ripe tomatoes, seeded and chopped into 1/4-inch pieces

DIRECTIONS:

1. Stir together the tomatoes, avocado, onion, lemon juice and Tabasco in a small bowl.
2. Season with salt and pepper to taste.
3. Mix the sour cream, coriander, salt and pepper in another small bowl to taste.
4. On a baking sheet, place the tortillas and brush the tops with oil.
5. Broil tortillas from 2 to 4 inches warm to golden pale.
6. Sprinkle with cheese and broil the tortillas uniformly until the cheese is melted.
7. To make 2 quesadillas, spread the avocado mixture evenly over two tortillas and cover each with 1 of the remaining tortillas, cheese side down.
8. Place the quesadillas on a cutting board; cut them into four wedges.
9. Top a dollop of the sour cream mixture with each wedge and serve soft.

Cheesy Chicken Salad

Prep Time: 35 minutes

Servings: 1-2

INGREDIENTS:

- 1 cup cooked chicken breast,cubed
- 1⁄4 cup carrot, shaved into ribbons
- 1⁄2 cup Baby Spinach, roughly chopped
- 1⁄4 cup celery, finely chopped
- 2 1⁄2 tablespoons fat-free mayonnaise
- 2 tablespoons nonfat sour cream
- 2 teaspoons Dijon mustard
- 1⁄8 teaspoon dried parsley
- 1⁄4 cup cheddar cheese, shredded

DIRECTIONS:

1. Mix all the ingredients in a bowl so that the mayonnaise mixture covers it well.
2. Chill for a minimum of 30 minutes in the fridge, but you should do it the night before.
3. Just serve.

Salad With Derby Dressing

Prep Time: 30 minutes

Servings: 2

INGREDIENTS:

- ½ bunch watercress
- ½ head iceberg lettuce
- 1 bunch chicory lettuce
- 2 medium tomatoes, skinned and seeded
- ½-pound smoked turkey breast
- ½ head romaine lettuce
- 6 slices crisp bacon
- 3 hard-boiled eggs
- 2 tablespoons chives chopped fine
- 1 avocado, sliced in half, seeded and peeled
- ½ cup blue cheese, crumbled

DRESSING:

- ⅛ teaspoon sugar
- ¾ teaspoon kosher salt
- 2 tablespoons water
- ½ teaspoon Worcestershire sauce
- 1 tablespoon fresh lemon juice
- ½ teaspoon fresh ground black pepper
- 2 tablespoons balsamic vinegar
- ⅛ teaspoon Dijon mustard
- 2 garlic cloves, minced very fine
- 2 tablespoons olive oil

DIRECTIONS:

1. Slice all the greens, very fine, very fine (almost minced).
2. Arrange them in rows in a bowl of chilled salad.
3. Break the tomatoes in half, seed them, and finely chop them.
4. Dice the ham, avocado, bacon and eggs.
5. Arrange the lettuce in rows with all the ingredients, including the blue cheese.
6. Sprinkle the chives on them.
7. Present in this manner at the table, then at the very last minute, toss with the dressing and serve in chilled salad bowls.
8. Serve with fresh French bread.

DRESSING:

1. Combine all the ingredients in a blender, except the olive oil and mix.
2. Add the oil slowly, with the machine going, and mix well.
3. Keep them refrigerated.

NOTE: This dish must be kept cool and eaten as cold as possible.

Pickled Onion

Prep Time: 25 minutes

Servings: 2

INGREDIENTS:

- 1 red onion, peeled, finely sliced
- 1 tablespoon sugar
- ¼ cup apple cider vinegar
- 1 teaspoon salt

DIRECTIONS:

1. To extract surplus moisture, pat the tofu with a few pieces of kitchen roll. I want them to be imperfect, not cubes because they look better! Use a knife to split the tofu into roughly 1-inch pieces.
2. Place the breadcrumbs in a shallow, large cup.
3. In another large, shallow cup, place the flour, salt, smoked paprika, cayenne and cumin and stir together.
4. Put the milk in a shallow bowl that is third deep.
5. Take the pieces of tofu and gently coat them on a baking sheet with the flour, then the milk, then the breadcrumbs.
6. Fill a deep-frying pan with vegetable oil about 1/2 inch deep. Put it over medium heat and let the oil get hot. To the oil, add chunks of breaded tofu and fry until golden underneath, then flip and cook so that it's all golden. Remove to a baking sheet lined with a drainable kitchen roll. Repeat with the tofu that remains.

For the pickled onion:

1. Heat the vinegar, salt and sugar from the apple cider in a small pot until steaming. In a bowl or pot, put the finely sliced red onion and pour the hot vinegar over it. To soften and turn pink, let it sit for at least 30 minutes.
2. Serve the spicy fried tofu, pickled onion, a smear of vegan mayo, some avocado and shredded cabbage in warmed tortillas (I warm them over my stove's lit gas ring).

Chicken Breasts With Avocado Tapenade

Prep Time: 15 minutes

Servings: 4

INGREDIENTS:

- 1 tablespoon grated lemon peel
- 4 boneless skinless chicken breast halves
- 5 tablespoons fresh lemon juice, divided
- 1 teaspoon olive oil, divided
- 1 garlic clove, finely chopped
- 2 tablespoons olive oil, divided
- 1⁄2 teaspoon salt
- 2 garlic cloves, roasted and mashed
- 1⁄2 teaspoon sea salt
- 1⁄4 teaspoon ground black pepper
- 1⁄4 teaspoon fresh ground pepper
- 1⁄4 cup small green pimento-stuffed olive, thinly sliced
- 3 tablespoons capers, rinsed
- 1 medium tomato, seeded and finely chopped
- 2 tablespoons fresh basil leaves, finely sliced
- 1 large Hass avocado, ripe, finely chopped

DIRECTIONS:

1. Combine the chicken and lemon peel marinade, 2 tablespoons of lemon juice, and 2 tablespoons of olive oil, salt, garlic, and pepper in a sealable plastic container. Seal the bag for 30 minutes and refrigerate.
2. Mix the remaining three tablespoons of lemon juice, roasted garlic, the remaining 1/2 teaspoon of olive oil, fresh ground pepper and sea salt in a bowl. Tomato, green olives, capers, basil, and avocado mixture; set aside.
3. Remove the bag of chicken and discard the marinade. Grill for 5 minutes on each side or to the optimum degree of cooking over medium-hot coals.
4. With Avocado Tapenade, serve.

LUNCH

Tilapia Parmesan

Prep Time: 35 minutes

Servings: 4

INGREDIENTS:
- 1/2 cup grated parmesan cheese
- 2 tablespoons lemon juice
- 3 tablespoons mayonnaise
- 3 tablespoons finely chopped green onions
- 4 tablespoons butter, room temperature
- 1/4 teaspoon dried basil
- 1 tablespoon black pepper
- 1/4 teaspoon seasoning salt
- 1 dash hot pepper sauce
- 2 pounds tilapia fillets

DIRECTIONS:
1. Preheat the oven to 350°C.
2. Lay the fillets in a single layer in a buttered 13-by-9-inch baking dish or jelly roll pan.
3. Do not have fillets stacked.
4. Brush with juice on top.
5. Mix the cheese, butter, mayonnaise, onions and seasonings in a dish.
6. Blend well with the fork.
7. In a preheated oven, bake the fish for 10 to 20 minutes or until the fish just begins to flake.
8. Spread with cheese mixture and bake for around 5 minutes, until golden brown.
9. Baking time will depend on the fish thickness that you are using.
10. Control the fish carefully so that they do not overcook.
    Note: You can make this fish in a broiler, too.
11. Broil for 3-4 minutes or until nearly through.
12. Attach the cheese and broil for 3 minutes or until it is browned.

Brussels Sprouts With Bacon And Onions

Prep Time: 30 minutes

Servings: 6

INGREDIENTS:

- 1 small yellow onion, thinly sliced
- 2 slices of bacon
- ¾ cup water
- 1 teaspoon Dijon mustard
- ¼ teaspoon salt
- 1 tablespoon cider vinegar
- 1 pound Brussels sprout, trimmed, halved and very thinly sliced

DIRECTIONS:

1. Cook bacon in a large pan until crisp 5 to 7 minutes over medium heat.
2. Transfer the onion and salt to the drippings in the pan, and cook over medium heat until tender and browned, frequently stirring (about 3 minutes).
3. Add water and mustard, scrape any browned parts, add sprouts from Brussels and cook, stirring regularly, until tender (4 to 6 minutes).
4. Stir in the vinegar and add the crumbled bacon to the tip.

Roasted Broccoli And Toasted Pine Nuts

Prep Time: 22 minutes

Servings: 4

INGREDIENTS:

- 1 pound broccoli floret
- Salt & freshly ground black pepper
- 2 tablespoons olive oil
- 2 tablespoons unsalted butter
- 1⁄2 teaspoon lemon zest, grated
- 1 teaspoon garlic, minced
- 1 -2 tablespoons fresh lemon juice
- 2 tablespoons pine nuts, toasted

DIRECTIONS:

1. Preheat the oven to 500°C.
2. Toss the broccoli with the oil in a wide bowl and add salt and pepper to taste.
3. On a baking sheet, arrange the florets into a single layer and roast.
4. Meanwhile, over medium heat, melt the butter in a small saucepan.
5. Apply the zest of garlic and lemon and heat for about 1 minute, stirring.
6. Let the lemon juice cool slightly and stir it in.
7. In a serving bowl, put the broccoli, pour the lemon butter and mix to coat it.
8. Over the top, scatter the toasted pine nuts.

Roasted Cauliflower

Prep Time: 1 hour 10 minutes

Servings: 4

INGREDIENTS:

- 4 tablespoons olive oil
- 1 head cauliflower or 1 equal head amount of pre-cut commercially prepped cauliflower
- 1 teaspoon salt, to taste

DIRECTIONS:

1. Preheat the oven to 425°C.
2. Trim the cauliflower head, discarding the thick stems and the core; cut the florets into pieces around the size of ping-pong balls.
3. Combine the olive oil and salt in a large bowl, whisk, then add the pieces of cauliflower and toss thoroughly.
4. For quick cleaning, line a baking sheet with parchment (you can skip that, if you don't have one then spread the pieces of cauliflower on the sheet and roast for 1 hour, turning three or four times, until most of each piece turns golden brown.
5. The browner the pieces of cauliflower turn; the more caramelization happens and the sweeter they taste.
6. Serve and drink it instantly!

Best Baked Potato

Prep Time: 1 hour 10 minutes

Servings: 1

INGREDIENTS:

- 2 tablespoons Canola oil
- 1 large russet potato
- Kosher salt

DIRECTIONS:

1. Heat the oven to 350°F and place the upper and lower thirds of the racks.
2. Thoroughly wash the potato (or potatoes) with a stiff brush and cold running water.
3. Dry, then poke 10 to 14 deep holes all over the spud using a regular fork so that moisture can escape during cooking.
4. Place it in a bowl and gently coat it with oil.
5. Sprinkle with kosher salt and put the potato in the middle of the oven directly on a rack.
6. To trap any drippings, place a baking sheet (I placed a piece of aluminum foil) on the lower rack.
7. Bake for 1 hour or until the skin feels crisp, but the flesh feels soft underneath.
8. Serve by forming a dotted line with your fork from end to end, then crack the spud open by pressing the ends towards each other.
9. It's going to pop open right.
10. But watch out, there's going to be some steam there.

NOTE: You will need to increase the cooking time by up to 15 minutes if you are cooking more than four potatoes.

Easy Black Bean Soup

Prep Time: 25 minutes

Servings: 4

INGREDIENTS:

- 3 tablespoons olive oil
- 1 tablespoon ground cumin
- 1 medium onion, chopped
- 2 -3 garlic cloves
- 2 (14 1/2 ounces) cans black beans
- Salt and pepper
- 2 cups chicken broth
- 1 small red onion
- ¼ cup cilantro, coarsely chopped

DIRECTIONS:

1. In olive oil, sauté the onion.
2. Add cumin when the onion becomes translucent.
3. Cook for 30 seconds, add garlic and cook for an additional 30 to 60 seconds.
4. Add 1 can of vegetable broth and 2 cups of black beans.
5. Bring to a boil, sometimes stirring.
6. Turn the heat off.
7. Mix the ingredients in the pot using a hand blender, or switch them to a blender.
8. Connect the second can of beans and the mixed ingredients to the pot and bring to a simmer.
9. Serve the soup with red onion bowls and cilantro for garnishing.
10. I'm also adding a bit of cilantro to the pot.
11. It can be doubled or frozen.

Vegan Lentil Burgers

Prep Time: 1 hour 10 minutes

Servings: 8-10 burgers

INGREDIENTS:

- 2 1⁄2 cups water
- 1 cup dry lentils, well rinsed
- 1⁄2 teaspoon salt
- 1⁄2 medium onion, diced
- 1 carrot, diced
- 1 tablespoon olive oil
- 1 teaspoon pepper
- 1 tablespoon soy sauce
- 3⁄4 cup breadcrumbs
- 3⁄4 cup rolled oats, finely ground

DIRECTIONS:

1. Boil the lentils with the salt in the water for about 45 minutes. The lentils are going to be soft, and much of the water is gone.
2. It will take about 5 minutes to fry the onions and carrots in oil until tender.
3. The cooked ingredients are combined in a bowl with pepper, soy sauce, oats, and bread crumbs.
4. While the mixture is still warm, it will produce ten burgers.
5. Burgers can then be fried shallowly on each side for 1-2 minutes or baked for 15 minutes at 200 C.

Coconut Kefir Banana Muffins

Prep Time: 45 minutes

Servings: 12

INGREDIENTS:

- 2 cups all-purpose flour
- 1 cup unsweetened dried shredded coconut
- 1 cup granulated sugar
- 2 teaspoons baking soda
- 1⁄2 teaspoon salt
- 2 ripe bananas, mashed
- 1 teaspoon baking powder
- 1⁄4 cup cold-pressed liquid coconut oil
- 1 1⁄2 cup pc dairy-free kefir probiotic fermented coconut milk
- 1 teaspoon vanilla extract

DIRECTIONS:

1. Preheat the oven to 180°C (350°F). Mist 12-Count Cooking Spray Muffin Tin. Only set aside.
2. In a big bowl, whisk together the flour, sugar, coconut, baking soda, baking powder and salt. Only set aside.
3. In a separate, large cup, whisk together the bananas, kefir, coconut oil and vanilla. Add to the flour mixture; stir until there are no white streaks left.
4. Divide the prepared muffin tin between the wells. Cook until the tops are golden and the toothpick inserted in the centers comes out clean, about 30 minutes. Let it cool for 15 minutes in the muffin pan.

   Chef's tip: let them cool fully on a rack to freeze muffins; you may individually cover the muffins in plastic wrap or foil before placing them in the container or bag for additional protection against freezer burn. Overnight in the oven, thaw muffins or microwave straight from frozen until warmed through around 20 to 30 seconds.

Sauerkraut Salad

Prep Time: 15 minutes

Servings: 6

INGREDIENTS:

- 1 cup celery, chopped fine
- 1 (1 pound) can sauerkraut, drained but not rinsed
- 1⁄2 cup green pepper, chopped fine
- 1⁄2 teaspoon salt
- 2 tablespoons onions, chopped fine
- 1⁄2 teaspoon pepper
- 1⁄3 cup salad oil
- 3⁄4 cup sugar
- 1⁄3 cup cider (I use white) or 1/3 cup white vinegar (I use white)

DIRECTIONS:

1. Mix the sauerkraut with the chopped vegetables.
2. On low heat, heat the sugar, oil, vinegar, salt and pepper until the sugar dissolves.
3. Refrigerate and pour over the vegetables.
4. Overnight relax.
5. Bake for 40-45 minutes at 350°F or until the top becomes crunchy.

Chocolate Keto Fat Bombs

Prep Time: 8 minutes

Servings:: 24

INGREDIENTS:

- 2/3 cup coconut oil
- 1/2 cup dark cocoa
- 4 (6 g) packets stevia
- 2/3 cup smooth peanut butter
- 1 tablespoon ground cinnamon
- 1/2 cup toasted coconut flakes
- 1/4 teaspoon kosher salt
- 1/4 teaspoon cayenne

DIRECTIONS:

1. In boiler set over a pot of hot water, blend the coconut oil, peanut butter, and cocoa powder. Heat, whisking, until smooth and molten.
2. To mix, add stevia, cinnamon, and salt and stir.
3. Divide the mixture into a mini muffin tray made of silicone. Top with coconut and cayenne and move to the freezer for about 30 minutes, until solid.

Breakfast Casserole

Prep Time: 12 minutes

Servings:: 6

INGREDIENTS:

- 2 pounds pork sausage
- 12 eggs
- 1 cup sour cream (light or regular)
- 1/4 cup milk
- Salt and pepper
- 4 green onions
- 1/2 green bell pepper, diced
- 1/2 red bell pepper, diced
- 2 cups shredded cheddar cheese

DIRECTIONS:

1. Preheat the oven to 350°C. Spray with cooking spray on a 9x13″ pan.

2. In a big bowl, mix the eggs, sour cream, milk, cheese, and salt and pepper. Mix with electric mixers at low speeds, only until mixed.

3. Over medium heat, heat a large skillet. Attach the sausage and cook until browned, breaking it with a wooden spoon into small pieces as it cooks. Drain much of the grease and use the egg mixture to add the sausage to the dish.

4. To the same pan, the sausage was cooked in, add the bell peppers and onion and sauté for 2-3 minutes. Add the eggs to the bowl and stir it to blend.

5. Pour the mixture into a 9x13″ greased pan and cook for 35-50 minutes or until the edges are set, and the middle is barely jiggly.

6. You can store the egg casserole in the fridge and enjoy it within 3-4 days. Leftovers reheated in the microwave are delicious.

NUTRITION:

Calories: 385 Kcal
Carbohydrates: 2 g
Sodium: 669 mg
Protein: 23 g
Fat: 30 g
Vitamin C: 11.6 mg
Saturated Fat: 12 g

Potassium: 327 mg
Sugar: 1 g
Vitamin A: 705 IU
Calcium: 194 mg
Cholesterol: 239 mg
Iron: 1.8 mg

Breakfast Burritos

Cook Time: 15 minutes

Prep Time: 25 minutes

Total Time: 40 minutes

Servings: 4

INGREDIENTS:

THE TOMATO-AVOCADO SALSA
- 1/2 cup diced seeded tomatoes, from 1 to 2 tomatoes
- 1/2 teaspoon salt
- 1 large avocado, pitted, peeled, and diced
- 1 garlic clove, minced
- 1 jalapeño pepper, seeded and minced
- 1 small shallot, minced (about 2 tablespoons)
- 1 tablespoon lime juice
- 1/4 teaspoon ground cumin
- 1/4 cup fresh chopped cilantro

FOR THE BURRITOS
- 4 large eggs
- 1/4 teaspoon salt
- 1/4 teaspoon smoked paprika
- 1-1/3 cup (6 ounces) shredded Monterey Jack cheese
- 4 (10-in) burrito-size flour tortillas
- Vegetable oil
- 1/2 pound spicy sausage (such as Italian, chorizo, or anything you like), removed from casings

DIRECTIONS:
1. Make the Avocado-Tomato Salsa: In a medium bowl, put all of the ingredients and blend to combine. Only set aside.
2. Whisk the eggs with the smoked paprika and salt in a medium dish. Only set aside.
3. Over medium-high heat, heat a large nonstick pan. Attach the sausage and cook for 4 to 5 minutes, often stirring, until it is browned. Move the sausage from the pan to a plate using a slotted spoon,

leaving the drippings in the pan. Lower the heat to a low level. Attach the eggs and scramble until they're ready to cook. Move to a plate with the eggs. Clean (you can need again the pan.

4. Assemble the burritos: Spoon on each tortilla about 1/4 cup of the avocado-salsa (you'll have a little leftover salsa; that's for the cook!), followed by a quarter of the bacon, a quarter of the eggs, and 1/3 cup of cheese. Fold over the filling on the sides of the tortilla and roll, tucking in the edges as you go.

5. Cover the pan lightly with oil and set over medium heat. Add the burritos, seam side down, when the pan is heated. Cook, covered until the burritos are golden brown at the rim, around 3 minutes. Flip the burritos over, and sealed, them until golden. Serve it sweet.

Make-Ahead: The burritos can be assembled before cooking a few hours ahead of time, securely wrapped in plastic wrap and refrigerated. Wrap in foil to reheat leftover burritos and warm for about 15 minutes in a 350°F oven.

Huevos Rancheros

Cook Time: 10 minutes

Prep Time: 5 minutes

Total Time: 15 minutes

INGREDIENTS:

- 2 large eggs
- 1/4 onion chopped
- 2 corn tortillas
- Refried beans homemade or store-bought
- Thick-cut ham cut into cubes
- Salsa - homemade or store-bought.
- 2 potatoes
- Salt and pepper to taste
- Fresh cheese and cilantro to garnish.

DIRECTIONS:

1. In a small amount of olive oil, sauté the potatoes, onion, and ham and season with salt and pepper to taste. Only set aside.
2. Fry the tortillas gently and pat them dry. Put yourself on a plate,
3. Heat the refried beans and scatter them over the tortillas.
4. Fry an egg and put it on top of the tortilla and beans at your desired level of doneness.
5. Round it off with salsa, fresh cheese, and fresh cilantro.
6. Serve with a combination of potatoes, onion, and ham.

Mexican Breakfast Casserole

Prep Time: 20 minutes

Cook Time: 55 minutes

Total Time: 75 minutes

Yield: 12 servings

INGREDIENTS:

- 1 small white onion, peeled and diced
- 1.25 pounds ground sausage* or Mexican chorizo
- 1 poblano or green bell pepper
- 1 (15-ounces) jar red or green salsa
- 4 garlic cloves, minced
- 1 (15-ounces) can black or pinto beans, rinsed and drained
- 1 teaspoon ground cumin
- 2/3 cup whole-kernel corn
- 1 teaspoon fine sea salt
- 12 large eggs
- 1/3 cup milk
- Eight corn tortillas halved
- Optional toppings: diced avocado, chopped fresh cilantro, diced red onion, diced green onion, or crumbled cotija cheese or sliced fresh jalapeños,
- 3 cups shredded Mexican-blend cheese

DIRECTIONS:

1. Heat the oven to 400°F.
2. In a large one, cook the sausage over medium heat until brown. To move the sausage to a clean plate, use a slotted spoon to reserve a tablespoon or so of grease in the saucepan. Add the onion and pepper and sauté, stirring periodically, until softened, for 5 minutes.
3. Attach the garlic and sauté, stirring periodically, until fragrant, for 1-2 minutes more. Apply the beans, corn, cumin, salt, and cooked sausage to the salsa, and stir until the mixture is thoroughly mixed.
4. Set aside and remove the pan from the heat. Mix the milk and eggs in a medium bowl.
5. Time to layer all the ingredients!

6. Spread half the tortillas on the bottom of the pan; now add half the chorizo, half the cheese and half the egg mixture. Repeat the tortillas, sausage mixture, egg mixture, and cheese with another layer. Cover the dish with foil and cook for 45-50 minutes, or until cooked through the middle of the casserole.

7. Move the baking dish to a rack for wire cooling and let it cool for 10 minutes.

8. Then sprinkle, slice and serve warm with your favorite toppings!

NOTES

Sausage: Any ground sausage of decent quality will fit well here! You might use bacon for breakfast, Italian sausage, Mexican chorizo, or whatever else you've got on hand. All will be perfect! Pork, beef, chicken or vegan sausage!

Cheesy Topping: If you want the cheese to be a little crispier on top of the casserole, just expose the casserole during the last 10 minutes of cooking.

Classic Hash Browns

Cook Time: 15 minutes

Prep Time: 5 minutes

Total Time: 20 minutes

Servings: 2

INGREDIENTS:

- 1/2 teaspoon salt
- 2 pounds Russet potatoes (4-5 small-to-medium, peeled)
- 1/2 teaspoon garlic powder
- 1/2 teaspoon paprika
- 1/4 cup vegetable oil
- 1/2 teaspoon onion powder

DIRECTIONS:

1. Scrub and clean the potatoes well then grate them on a large-holed grater of cheese.
2. On a fine-mesh sieve, arrange the potatoes, and cover them.
3. After putting them on a clean tea towel, drain the potatoes very well and press another towel on them to remove any residual moisture. It is important to extract as much moisture as possible.
4. In a wide bowl, pass the potatoes and if desired, toss with the salt, garlic powder, onion powder, paprika and some black pepper.
5. Place a large cast-iron pan over medium heat and add the oil once warm, heat it until it begins to shimmer, and if a piece of rubbed potato sizzles is added on contact.
6. In ONE LAYER, add the grated potatoes to the hot oil, press them down slightly and fry them unwaveringly for about 2 minutes to make them crispy and golden-brown.
7. For another 2 minutes, stir, press and cook. Repeat as needed, about 6 - 8 more minutes.
8. Move the cooked hash browns to a plate lined with paper towels and allow the excess oil to drain. Cook the remaining potatoes, meanwhile.
9. With a runny egg on top, serve sweet.

NUTRITION:

Calories: 299 Kcal

Carbohydrates: 41 g

Sugar: 1 g

Protein: 4 g

Fat: 13 g

Saturated Fat: 11 g

Cholesterol: 0 mg

Sodium: 302 mg

Potassium: 945 mg

Fiber: 3 mg

Calcium: 29 mg

Vitamin A: 125 IU

Vitamin C: 13 mg

Iron: 2 mg

DINNER

Zucchini And Eggs With Cheese

Cook Time: 16 minutes

Prep Time: 4 minutes

Total Time: 20 minutes

Servings: 1

INGREDIENTS:

- 1 yellow onion small, sliced thinly, about 4 ounces
- 1 tablespoon olive oil separated
- 2-3 garlic cloves sliced in half
- 1 small zucchini chopped into ½-inch quarters, about 6 ounces
- 1 egg room temperature, slightly beaten
- Salt and pepper to taste
- 1 tablespoon water
- 1 tablespoon Italian parsley chopped
- 1-2 tablespoons Romano cheese grated

DIRECTIONS:

1. Heat 1/2 tablespoon of olive oil over medium-high heat in a large skillet.
2. Add the onion and reduce to medium heat.
3. Cook, stirring until translucent periodically and softened for around 3-5 minutes.
4. The remaining chopped zucchini, olive oil, and garlic are added. With salt and pepper, season.
5. Sauté, stirring and shaking the pan, until golden brown, over medium-high heat. It should take about 7-10 minutes for this. The zucchini needs to be baked, but it's still crisp—a taste of doneness. If necessary, change the heat.
6. Meanwhile, whisk the cheese and parsley with the egg.
7. Add the egg mixture to the pan when the zucchini is cooked, and let it cook for about 30 seconds. Then stir and shake the pan until the egg is scrambled and set, for 1 minute or so.
8. Taste the seasonings and change.

9. Immediately serve.

10. Garnish with chopped Italian parsley and grated cheese, if needed.

NUTRITION:

Carbohydrates: 17 g

Calories: 280 Kcal

Protein: 10 g

Fat: 20 g

Saturated Fat: 4 g

Sodium: 141 mg

Potassium: 529 mg

Cholesterol: 169 mg

Fiber: 3 g

Sugar: 8 g

Iron: 2 mg

Vitamin A: 811 IU

Vitamin C: 36 mg

Calcium: 133 mg

Egg Scramble With Sweet Potatoes

Cook Time: 25 minutes

Prep Time: 5 minutes

Total Time: 30 minutes

Servings: 2

INGREDIENTS:

- 1/2 cup chopped onion
- 1 (8-ounce) sweet potato, diced
- 2 tsp chopped rosemary
- Salt
- 4 large eggs
- 4 large egg whites
- Pepper
- 2 tablespoons chopped chive

DIRECTIONS:

1. Preheat the heater to 425°F. Toss the sweet potato, onion, rosemary, and salt and pepper into a baking dish. Spray with cooking spray and roast for about 20 minutes.
2. Meanwhile, whisk the eggs, egg whites, and a pinch of salt and pepper together in a medium cup. Spritz a cooking spray skillet and scramble the eggs over medium heat for around 5 minutes.
3. Sprinkle and serve with the spuds with chopped chives.

NUTRITION:

Calories per serving: 571 Kcal

Protein: 44 g

Carbohydrates: 52 g

Fiber: 9 g

Fat: 20 g

Spicy Tomato Baked Eggs

Cook Time: 25 minutes

Prep Time: 5 minutes

Total Time: 30 minutes

Servings: 2

INGREDIENTS:

- 1 tablespoon olive oil
- 1 red pepper
- 2 red onions, peeled and cut into half-moons
- 1 garlic clove, peeled and sliced
- 1 teaspoon paprika
- 4 medium eggs
- 250 g cherry tomatoes, halved or 1 tin peeled plum tomatoes
- 2 tablespoons chopped flat-leaf parsley (optional)

DIRECTIONS:

1. Preheat the oven to 180 /Gas 6 200°C/fan.
2. Heat the oil in an frying pan.
3. Add the onions, garlic and pepper. Season with ground black pepper and cook until soft or for 10 minutes.
4. Add the tomatoes and paprika and cook gently for an additional 5 minutes.
5. In the mixture, make four little wells and crack an egg into each. Season, cover, and place in the oven with black pepper.
6. Cook until the eggs are set - this should take 5-8 minutes or so. If used, sprinkle over the parsley.

Vegetable Meatloaf

Cook Time: 20 minutes

Prep Time: 5 minutes

Total Time: 25 minutes

Servings: 2

INGREDIENTS:

- 2 tablespoons extra-virgin olive oil
- 1 small zucchini, finely diced
- 1 large egg, lightly beaten
- 1 red bell pepper, finely diced
- 1 yellow bell pepper, finely diced
- 5 garlic cloves smashed to a paste with coarse salt
- Kosher salt and freshly ground pepper
- 1/4 cup chopped fresh parsley
- 1/2 cup Parmesan cheese or freshly grated Romano
- 1 1/2 pound ground turkey
- 1 cup panko (coarse Japanese breadcrumbs)
- 1 tablespoon finely chopped fresh thyme
- 1/4 cup plus 2 tablespoons balsamic vinegar
- 3/4 cup ketchup

DIRECTIONS:

1. Preheat the oven to 425°F. Over high pressure, heat the oil in a large sauté pan. Add the zucchini, garlic paste, bell peppers, and 1/4 teaspoon of red pepper flakes. Season with pepper and salt and cook for about 5 minutes, until the vegetables are almost tender. Set to cool aside.

2. In a large cup, whisk in the egg and fresh herbs. Add turkey, panko, grated cheese, 1/2 cup of ketchup, 2 tablespoons of cooled vegetables and balsamic vinegar; blend until just mixed.

3. Press the mixture into a 9-by-5-inch loaf pan gently. In a small bowl, whisk 1/4 cup balsamic vinegar and 1/4 cup ketchup, and 1/4 teaspoon red pepper flakes; brush the blend over the whole loaf. For 1 to 1 1/4 hours, bake. Until slicing, let it rest for 10 minutes.

133

Easy Bbq Chicken Toasts

Prep Time: 10 minutes

Total Time: 18 minutes

Cook Time: 8 minutes

Servings: 4

INGREDIENTS:

- 3 cups cooked and shredded chicken
- 1 1/2 cup of your favorite barbecue sauce, divided
- 8 tostada shells or eight corn tortillas, coated with olive oil and baked for 5 minutes per side
- 3 green onions, very thinly sliced
- 2 cups shredded cheese

DIRECTIONS:

1. Preheat to 350°F in your oven. Spread out 2 rimmed baking sheets with the tostada shells (or baked tortillas).
2. In a medium bowl, mix the chicken and 1 cup of barbecue sauce, and swirl to coat.
3. Divide the chicken between the shells of the tostada and top with the cheese (approximately ¼ cup each).
4. Bake, only until the cheese is melted, for 6 to 8 minutes.
5. Remove and drizzle with the remaining ½ cup of barbecue sauce from the oven. If needed, sprinkle it with green onions.

NUTRITION:

Serving: 2 toasts

Vitamin A: 825 IU

Calories: 693 kcal

Carbohydrates: 66 g

Protein: 31 g

Fat: 33 g

Saturated Fat: 13 g

Sodium: 1730 mg

Potassium: 554 mg

Fiber: 3 g

Sugar: 36 g

Vitamin C: 3.7 mg

Calcium: 359 mg

Cholesterol: 107 mg

Iron: 2.3 mg

Buffalo Chicken Sandwich With Cheese

Cook Time: 20 minutes

Prep Time: 10 minutes

Total Time: 30 minutes

Servings: 2

INGREDIENTS:

Blue Cheese Slaw:

- 1/4 cup mayonnaise
- 1 tablespoon minced garlic
- 1/4 cup crumbled blue cheese
- 2 tablespoons Worcestershire sauce
- 1 (10-ounce) package coleslaw mix
- Kosher salt
- 1 lemon, juiced
- Freshly cracked black pepper
- Canola oil, to fry

Buffalo Chicken:

- 1/2 cup buffalo hot sauce, store-bought
- 2 tablespoons smoked paprika
- 4 (6-ounce) boneless, skinless chicken cutlets
- 1 tablespoon kosher salt
- 1 cup self-rising flour
- 1 1/4 cups buttermilk
- 2 tablespoons hot sauce
- 1 egg
- 1 tablespoon cracked black pepper
- 4 soft-club rolls, split and toasted

DIRECTIONS:

1. Mix the mayonnaise, garlic, crumbled blue cheese Worcestershire sauce, and lemon juice in a medium-sized bow. Attach the mix of coleslaw and toss well. With salt and pepper, season and set aside.

2. Heat enough canola oil in a deep-fryer or heavy-bottomed pot to get halfway up the sides of the pot, to 350°F.

3. In a shallow dish, add buffalo sauce and set aside. To taste, season the chicken with smoked paprika and salt and pepper. In a shallow dish, place the flour, 2 tablespoons of paprika, 1 tablespoon of salt and 1 tablespoon of pepper. Put the egg, buttermilk, and hot sauce together in another shallow dish and whisk together. Dredge each piece of chicken and shake off any excess in the buttermilk mixture, then dredge it into the flour mixture. Fry until the chicken is cooked through around 4 to 6 minutes, and on an instant-read thermometer, the internal temperature registers 165°F. In the buffalo sauce, dip the finished chicken and place it on the club rolls. Top the chicken and shape a sandwich with a liberal quantity of slaw.

Italian Chicken

Cook Time: 30 minutes

Prep Time: 10 minutes

Total Time: 40 minutes

Servings: 2

INGREDIENTS:

- 4 boneless skinless chicken breasts
- 1/2 cup breadcrumbs
- 1/2 cup grated parmesan cheese
- 1/2 teaspoon minced garlic
- Salt and pepper to taste
- 4 tablespoons butter melted
- 1 teaspoon Italian seasoning
- 1-pound small potatoes halved or quartered
- Cooking spray
- 2 tablespoons chopped parsley
- Lemon wedges optional garnish

DIRECTIONS:

1. To 400°F, preheat the oven. Using cooking spray to cover a sheet pan.
2. Mix the parmesan cheese, breadcrumbs, garlic, Italian seasoning, salt and pepper together in a small cup.
3. In the melted butter, dip the top of each chicken breast,
4. On the prepared sheet pan, put the chicken breasts.
5. About the chicken, scatter the potatoes. Drizzle over the potatoes and chicken with the remaining butter. With salt and pepper, season the potatoes.
6. Bake for 30 minutes or until the chicken is completely cooked and the potatoes are tender. Depending on the thickness of your chicken, the cooking time can vary.
7. Sprinkle and serve with parsley. If needed, garnish with lemon wedges.

NUTRITION:

Carbohydrates: 10 g

Calories: 336 Kcal

Protein: 32 g

Fat: 19 g

Saturated Fat: 11 g

Cholesterol: 113 mg

Vitamin A: 490 IU

Potassium: 460 mg

Vitamin C: 1.3 mg

Sodium: 520 mg

Calcium: 172 mg

Iron: 1.2 mg

Oriental Turkey Burgers

Cook Time: 30 minutes

Prep Time: 10 minutes

Total Time: 40 minutes

Servings: 2

INGREDIENTS:

SLAW

- 2 cups coleslaw mix
- 1 tablespoon seasoned rice vinegar
- 3 tablespoons chopped fresh cilantro
- 1 teaspoon vegetable oil

BURGER

- 2 tablespoons Butter
- 2 jalapeño chili peppers, seeded, finely chopped

- 1/3 cup chopped green onions
- 1 1/4 pound lean ground turkey
- 1 tablespoon hoisin sauce
- 1 tablespoon soy sauce
- 1/4 cup dry bread crumbs
- 1 tablespoon butter, melted
- Hoisin sauce, if desired
- 5 (10-inch) tortillas

DIRECTIONS:

1. Heat the gas grill until the coals are ash-white on a medium or charcoal grill.
2. In a tub, mix all the slaw ingredients; mix well. Cover; leave to cool before serving time.
3. Melt 2 tablespoons of butter until sizzling in a 10-inch skillet; add the onion and chili peppers. Cook for approximately 1-2 minutes or until tender. Cool.
4. In a cup, combine the onion mix, turkey, bread crumbs, 1 tablespoon of hoisin sauce and soy sauce; mix gently. Shape into four patties (3/4 inches thick).
5. Set the patties on the grill—with a molten butter brush. Grill, rotating once, for 20-30 minutes or until the inner temperature reaches a minimum of 165°F and the middle of the meat is no longer pink.
6. Wrap the aluminum foil tortillas. Place them away from direct heat on the grill. Move tortillas often when grilling burgers.
7. Place half of each warm tortilla with the burgers. Top with slaw; drizzle, if necessary, with hoisin sauce. Fold your tortilla over your burger.

Conclusion

Thanks for making it through to the end of this book, let's hope it was informative and able to provide you with all of the tools you need to achieve your goals whatever they may be.

One Meal A Day routine is a powerful technique to shed the extra weight and bring your fat under control. It is a systematic process through which you can easily lead a healthy and fit life.

This book has tried to explain not only the basics of the One Meal a Day routine but also the correct way to incorporate it into your life. The key to success in this routine is to remain patient and follow the steps correctly. You must not rush the process and always keep the basics in mind.

Following quick fixes for losing weight may give you results in the short term but they can never last long and such methods have their own side effects. One Meal a Day routine is safe, reliable and very effective. You only need to follow it with patience and perseverance.

You can also get all the benefits of the process by following the simple steps given in the book. I hope that this book is really able to help you in achieving your health goals.

Finally, if you found this book useful in any way, a review on Amazon is always appreciated!

Made in United States
North Haven, CT
02 January 2023

30415688R10078